Feline Anatomy
A Coloring Atlas

Robert A. Kainer, DVM, MS
Professor of Anatomy
Ross University
Basseterre, St. Kitts
West Indies

Thomas O. McCracken PhD Hon., MS, MS
Professor and Course Director Gross Anatomy
University of Medicine and Health Sciences
International University of Nursing
Basseterre, St. Kitts
West Indies

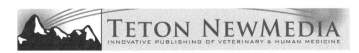
TETON NEWMEDIA
INNOVATIVE PUBLISHING OF VETERINARY & HUMAN MEDICINE

Jackson, Wyoming

Executive Editor: Carroll C. Cann
Layout: 5640 Design Inc., www.fiftysixforty.com
Illustrations by Thomas O. McCracken and David Carlson

Printed in the United States of America

Teton NewMedia
P.O. Box 4833
Jackson, WY 83001

1-888-770-3165
www.tetonnm.com

The authors and publishers have made every effort to provide an accurate reference text. However, they shall not be held responsible for problems arising from errors or omissions, or from misunderstandings on the part of the reader.

ISBN# 1-59161-045-1

Print Number 5 4 3 2 1

Library of Congress Cataloging-in-Publication Data on file

Table of Contents

Respiratory System

Urinary System

Female Reproductive System

Male Reproductive System

Nervous System

Endocrine System

Index

Acknowledgments

The authors express their gratitude to anatomy professors Dr. Anna Fails and Dr. Michael Smith for their critical review of the drawings and text. This input assisted substantially in the preparation of this atlas.

The patience and counsel of the staff at Teton NewMedia is gratefully acknowledged.

Several illustrations were redrawn from the following sources:

Hudson, Lola; Hamilton, William; *Atlas of Feline Anatomy for Veterinarians,* W.B. Saunders Company, 1993.

McCracken, T.; Kainer, R.: *Color Atlas of Small Animal Anatomy; The Essentials,* Blackwell Publishing, 2008.

Schneck, Marcus; Caravan, Jill; *Cat Facts,* Barnes & Noble Books, 2000.

The following publications were used for general reference:

Boyd, J.S.: *A Color Atlas of Clinical Anatomy of the Dog and Cat,* London, Mosby-Wolfe, 1991.

Crouch, J.; Atlas of Cat Anatomy, Lea and Febiger, 1969.

Done, S.H, Evans, S.A.; Strickland, N.C.: *Color Atlas of Veterinary Anatomy, Vol. 3, The Dog and Cat,* London, Mosby-Wolfe, 1996.

Gilbert, S., *Pictorial Anatomy of The Cat, Revised Edition,* University of Washington, 1975.

Popesko, P.: *Atlas of Topographical Anatomy of the Domestic Animals,* Philadelphia, W. B. Saunders, 1979.

Introduction

This coloring atlas was produced for those with a genuine interest in cats. The format is designed for the cat owner who desires to gain a basic knowledge of feline anatomy with functional correlations and brief descriptions of some of the diseases of the region being studied. Cat breeders, trainers and cat-show judges and students of veterinary medicine, veterinary medical technology, zoology and wildlife biology will find the contents useful for an initial background from which more detailed references can be pursued. Active learning is involved as you color anatomical structures and their names on the drawings or underline their names in the text and color the parts indicated by a corresponding number. Guiding symbols such as arrows or lines are also colored. As you color, the size, shape and position of organs and their relationships are made clear.

The cat, *Felis domestica* (*Genus species*), is a mammal in the Order Carnivora and Family Felidae. All cats, from the savage hunters of the plains and forest to the domestic pet are recognizably related. Most experts agree that there are 38 species of cats including the domestic cat. Domestic cats have a common ancestor, the African wild cat (*Felis libyca*). This cat inhabited most of Asia and North Africa, a lithely-built animal much like the tabby domestic cat. Close relatives of the cat due to similarities in skull structure are the mongoose, civet, and hyena.

Some physical characteristics of felidae:
  Prominent canine and premolar teeth for holding and cutting skin and flesh.
  Carnassial (shearing) teeth – lower 1st molar and upper 4th premolar teeth.
  A relatively short digestive tract.
  Anal sacs lined with sebaceous (oil) glands.
  Reproductive system producing several offspring in one gestation.
  Heart, lungs and muscular appendages adapted for running or digging.
  Retractable claws.

Today there are about 100 pedigree breeds recognized, Persians being the most popular. Nonpedigree cats, the majority of domestic cats, are referred to as moggie. Cats come in many different sizes, shapes and hair coats, cats fall into three main body types; cobby, muscular, and foreign. No matter the size, shape, or color, the basic anatomy and physiology are the same. In this atlas, you will explore the anatomy of the domestic cat and some of the variations among the different breeds.

The Authors

Thomas O. McCracken PhD Hon., MS, MS
Professor Anatomy and Physiology
University of Medicine and Health Sciences
International University of Nursing
PO Box 1218
Basseterre, St. Kitts
West Indies

Professor McCracken attended graduate school at the University of Michigan, receiving master's degrees in anatomy, physiology, and medical illustration. He was hired by Colorado State University as Director of Biomedical Media in the College of Veterinary Medicine and Biomedical Sciences. During the period from 1978 to 1985, he illustrated five major veterinary medical textbooks and over 75 scientific papers. In 1985, he was appointed to the faculty of the Department of Anatomy and Neurobiology as associate professor, and in 1990, he became director of the sixth accredited medical illustration program in the United States, and the only one associated with a veterinary medical school. Professor McCracken is currently course coordinator for gross and developmental anatomy at the university of Medicine and Health Sciences, St. Kitts. Over the years, Dr. McCracken has won numerous awards of excellence from the Association of Medical Illustrators for his anatomic and surgical illustrations. In 1997, he was the recipient of the Frank Netter Award for Special Contributions to Medical Education.

Robert A. Kainer, DVM, MS
Professor of Anatomy
Ross University
Basseterre, St. Kitts
West Indies

After receiving his DVM degree from Colorado A & M College (now CSU) in 1949, Dr. Kainer spent a summer at the University of Idaho, then four years at Washington State University where he taught anatomy and pursued graduate study in anatomy and pathology. For the next two years, he taught at Oklahoma State University. He returned to Colorado in 1955 to enter private veterinary practice in Idaho Springs. In 1961, he joined the anatomy faculty at Colorado State University. Among the honors he received during his 27 years at Colorado State are the Top Prof Award and the Oliver Pennock Award for teaching and scholarship at CSU, the Norden award for distinguished teaching in the field of veterinary medicine, and the Colorado Veterinary Medical Association 1986 Faculty of the Year Award. Dr. Kainer contributed his expertise in collaborative research on various veterinary medical problems, leading to over 60 publications.

How to Use this Coloring Atlas

Using this atlas, you will explore the cat's body by coloring drawings of its various organs and reading the short descriptions accompanying the drawings. Coloring illustrations in this manner is an enjoyable and effective learning experience. In keeping with the current trend in naming parts of the body, most Latin anatomic names have been changed to English.

Drawings of **organs** making up the **systems** of the cat's body are presented in plates. Pages opposite the plates contain directions for labeling and coloring the drawings. Essential anatomic and physiologic concepts are explained and some diseases common to the region being studied are discussed. Important terms are underlined in the text.

The atlas may be used alone, or it may be used to assist in dissection. The drawings on many of the plates represent prosected specimens. For the most part, each plate is self-contained, so the plates do not have to be studied in sequence. You may select the plates you wish to color first or to review later.

Before beginning, read the following important directions:
1. Look over the entire plate on the right page, and then read instructions for labeling and coloring on the left page. The names of structures to be colored are printed in **boldface type** preceded by numbers or letters that correspond with the numbers or letters on the plate.

2. Underline the words in **boldface type** on the left page in different colors, and use the same colors on the indicated structures, arrows or dashed lines on the drawings. Also underline or color over the terms labeling structures on the drawings and color the structures where appropriate.

3. The choice of colors is yours. Colored pencils or felt-tipped pens are recommended. Suggested coloring materials include Crayola© Washable Markers, Pentel© Color Pens, colored artists pencils, or similar media. Very dark colors obscure detail, so use lighter shades of these colors and test the colors before using them.

Surface of the Body

Regions of the Feline's Body

PLATE 1

Underline the names of the body's regions in different colors and, in matching colors, fill in the regions indicated on the drawing. You will probably have to go through your set of colors three or four times.

1. Pinna
2. Throatlatch
3. Commissure of lips
4. Flew
5. Nose
6. Muzzle
7. Foreface
8. Stop
9. Crown
10. Occiput
11. Crest
12. Neck
13. Withers
14. Shoulder

15. Point of shoulder
    (at the shoulder joint)
16. Chest
17. Arm
18. Elbow
19. Forearm
20. Carpus
21. Metacarpus (pastern)
22. Digits (toes of the forepaw)
    1,2,3,4,5
23. Back
24. Thorax
25. Loin
26. Abdomen (belly)

27. Flank
28. Point of hip
29. Croup (rump)
30. Set of tail
31. Buttock
32. Thigh
33. Stifle
34. Leg
35. Tarsus (hock)
36. Metatarsus (pastern)
37. Dewclaw (digit 1)

The region called **manus** (Latin for hand) is a human term and includes the carpus, metacarpus and digits.
The region called **pes** (Latin for foot) includes the tarsus, metatarsus and digits.
A **dewclaw** is a variably present first digit on the <u>hindlimb</u>. The term is commonly used to name the always present (but reduced) first digit on the forelimb.
The **trunk** includes all regions of the body exclusive of the head and limbs.

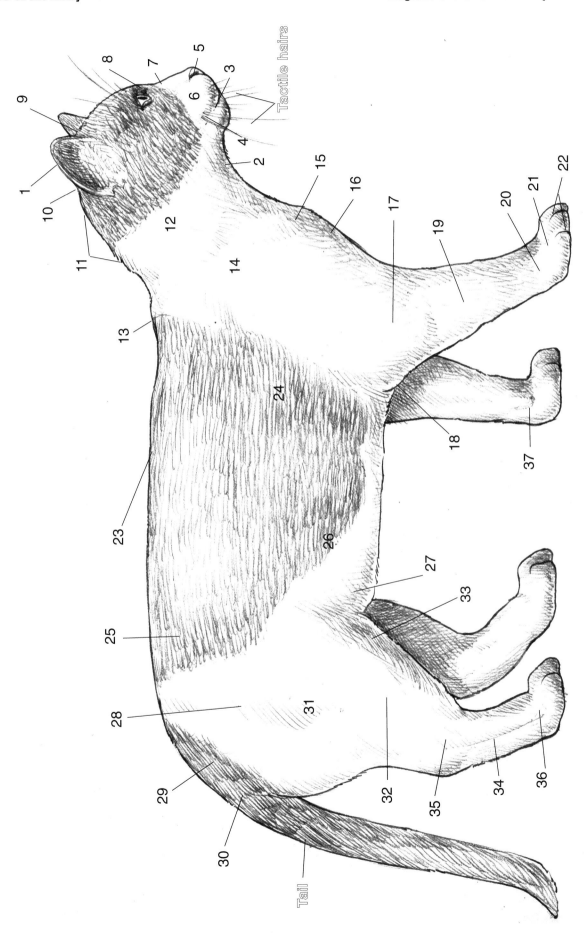

Tactile hairs

Tail

1
2
3
4
5
6
7
8
9
10
11
12
13
14
15
16
17
18
19
20
21
22
23
24
25
26
27
28
29
30
31
32
33
34
35
36
37

Directional Terms

PLATE 2

Directional terms (names) describe the locations of body parts, related functional changes in position, and define the extent of lesions (diseased regions). Color the words, arrows and dashed lines in matching colors.

Dorsal and **ventral** are opposite terms indicating the relative locations of parts toward the back, (Latin, *dorsum*) or the belly (L., *venter*). Above the carpus (wrist) and above the tarsus (hock) and from the belly to the back, a structure located close to the cranium (skull case) is **cranial** to another structure. A structure located toward the tail (L., *cauda*) is **caudal** to another.

On the head the term, **rostral**, is used to indicate the location of a part closer to the nose (L., *rostrum*). Caudal remains the same. **Proximal** indicates a location toward the attached end of a limb, closer to the trunk of the body. Proximal is also used to indicate a part of the alimentary canal toward the mouth.

Oral is a synonym. **Distal** indicates a location toward the free end of a limb, that is, farther from the trunk. Distal is also used to indicate a part of the alimentary canal away from the mouth. **Aboral** is a synonym.

Distal to and including the carpus, **dorsal** replaces cranial and **palmar** replaces caudal. Distal to and including the tarsus, **dorsal** replaces cranial and **plantar** replaces caudal.

On a frontal view of the distal end of a cat's limb, the **axis** is shown by a dashed line. An **axial** position is located toward the axis; an **abaxial** position, away from the axis.

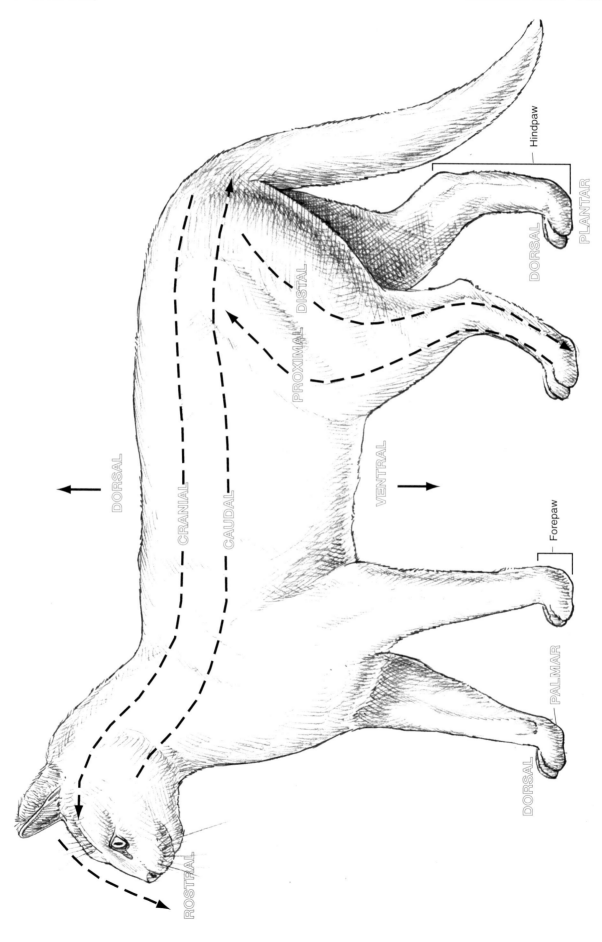

Body Planes

PLATE 3

Body planes are formed by any two points that can be connected by a straight line.

Fill in words, arrows, and dashed lines in different colors. Color the four body plane panels very lightly.

Figure 1. The **median plane** (L., *medianus* = in the middle), indicated by dashed lines between the m's, divides the cat's body into right and left halves. A **sagittal plane** (L., *sagitta* = arrow), indicated by the dashed line from s to s, is any plane parallel to the median plane.

Figure 2. The **median plane** is indicated by a dashed line. **Medial** and **lateral** (L., *latus* = flank) are directional terms relative to the median plane. Medial structures are "inside", located closer to the median plane. Lateral structures are "outside", away from the median plane, that is, toward the flank or side.

Figure 3. A **transverse plane**, indicated by a dashed line between the t's, passes through the head, trunk or limb perpendicular to the long axis of the part. A **horizontal plane (dorsal plane)**, indicated by a dashed line from d to d, passes through a body part parallel to its dorsal surface.

Figure 1

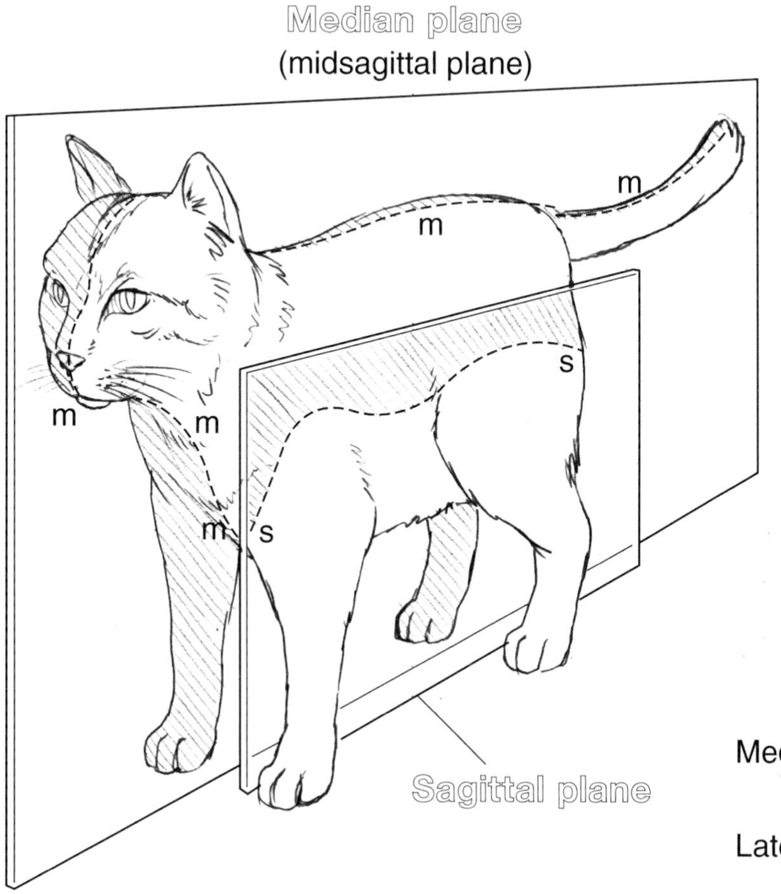

Median plane
(midsagittal plane)

m

m

m

m

s

m   s

Sagittal plane

Figure 2

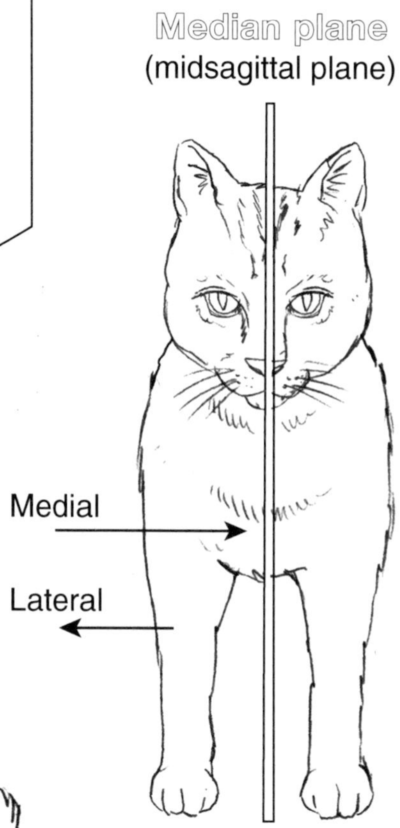

Median plane
(midsagittal plane)

Medial

Lateral

Figure 3

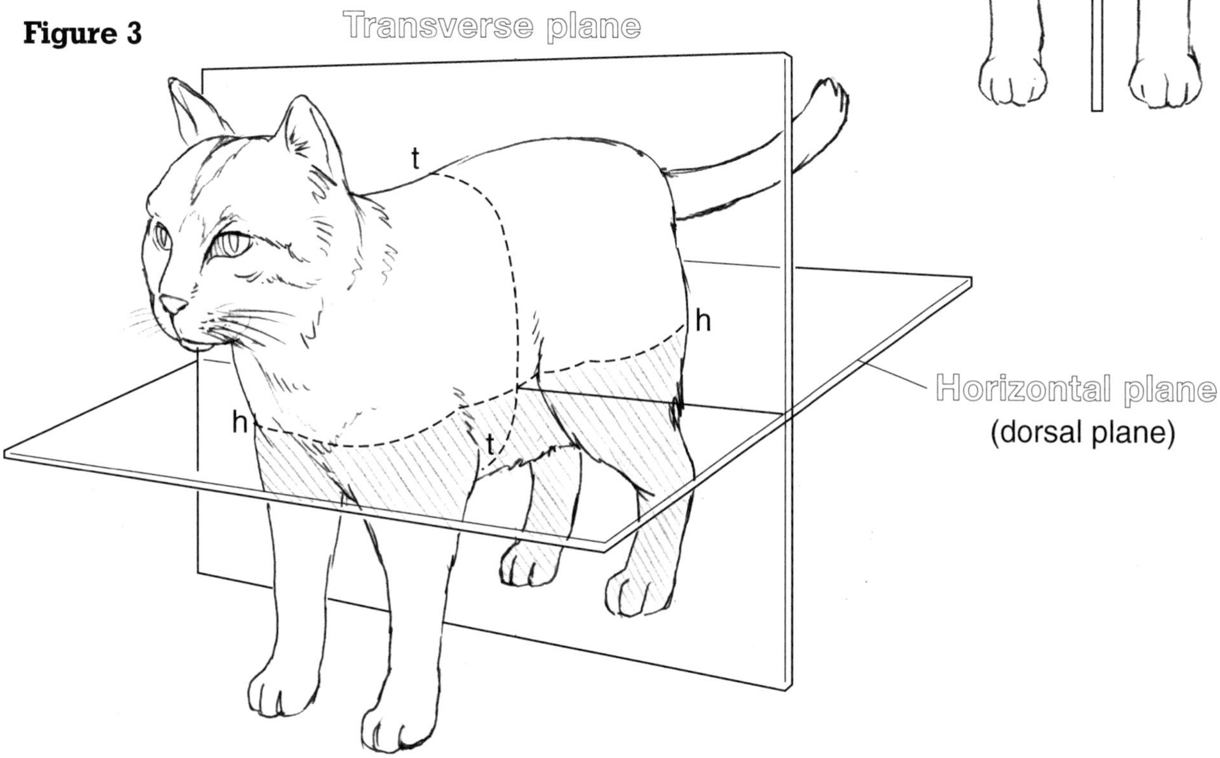

Transverse plane

t

h

h

t

Horizontal plane
(dorsal plane)

Anatomy of Feline Skin

PLATE 4

Prominent hair elevator muscles in the cat's skin elevate the hairs to trap air, providing insulation when outside temperature is cold. These muscles elevate the hairs highest when the cat is frightened or angry. Hair elevator muscles also squeeze oil glands that secrete into hair follicles. Apocrine sweat glands also open into hair follicles just superficial to the openings of the oil glands.

Figure 1. Large arrector pili muscles (hair elevator muscles)

Figure 2. Tactile hair (sinus hair)

Figure 3. Section of a foot pad: includes the stratum corneum, a thick horny layer in the epidermis, a dense fibrous layer (dermis) and subcutaneous tissue, containing fat cells, loose connective tissue, blood vessels, nerves and merocrine sweat glands that empty on the surface.

Figure 1

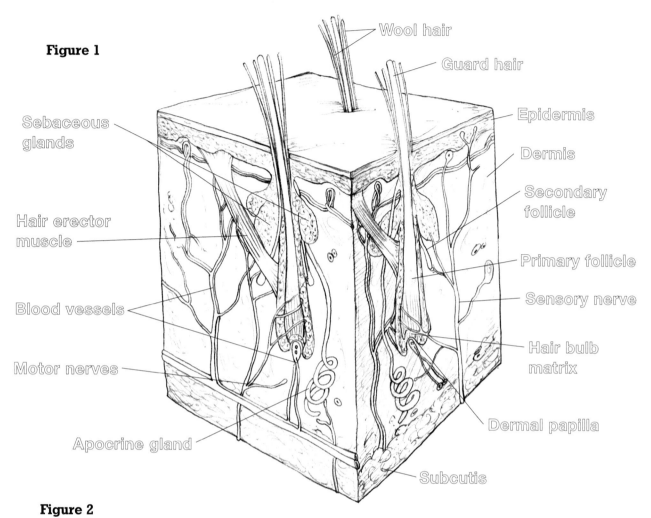

Wool hair

Guard hair

Epidermis

Dermis

Secondary follicle

Primary follicle

Sensory nerve

Hair bulb matrix

Dermal papilla

Subcutis

Sebaceous glands

Hair erector muscle

Blood vessels

Motor nerves

Apocrine gland

Figure 2

Figure 3

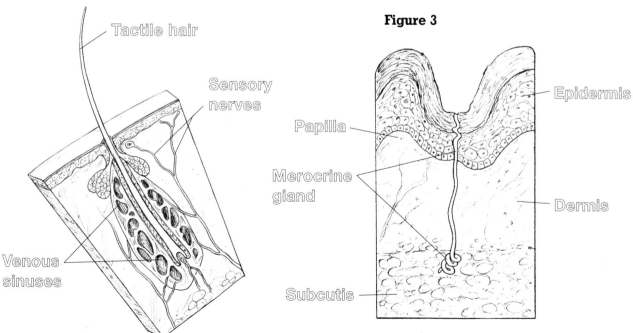

Tactile hair

Sensory nerves

Venous sinuses

Papilla

Merocrine gland

Subcutis

Epidermis

Dermis

Functions of Feline Skin

PLATE 5

The skin is the largest organ in the body - 11%-25% of body weight, being highest in kittens. As a sensory organ, its nerve endings provide information to the central nervous system on pressure, tension, pain, itching, and temperature. Color the names and structures indicated.

Figure 1. Section (slice) of feline skin. Higher magnification.
Keratinocytes (cells of the epidermis) multiply in the **basal layer** of the tissue. They change shape, becoming flat and cornified (horny) as they are moved to the **cornified layer (stratum corneum)** where they die. This process takes about three weeks. The cornifed, flat, dead cells remain in the layers of the stratum corneum for another three weeks before they are shed. Millions of surface cells shed each day.

In contact with the environment, the skin serves as a barrier to intrusion by living things (viruses, bacteria and larger parasites) and by physical and chemical agents. Protection is afforded by the cornified, dead, surface cells of the epidermis and by white blood cells and other immune system cells in the dermis. Water resistance is furnished by the surface cells of the epidermis, the dense hairs of the undercoat, and the oily sebum produced by the sebaceous glands.

The skin lends flexible support to underlying structures, and the subcutis lets the skin glide over them. This arrangement permits the skin to be shaken from side to side and recoil (as when shaking off water) without the cat losing balance. When a cat is dehydrated, the skin snaps back slowly when it is pinched and released.

Regulation of body temperature is aided by the skin. Blood vessels in the dermis and subcutis contract to reduce blood volume near the surface, thus conserving body heat. In a hot environment, blood vessels expand, bringing more blood near the surface to give off heat. The cat's apocrine tubular (sweat) glands produce only a scant, thick secretion that does not wet the skin as does the sweat of horses and people. Blood pressure control is assisted through contraction and expansion of blood vessels in the dermis and subcutis.

Figure 2. Hair cycle.
Production of hair is a joint task between a **dermal papilla** and a **hair bulb matrix**. The hair cycle includes an actively growing stage **(anagen)** followed by a stage **(catagen)** during which the hair bulb matrix sort of shrinks and peels away from its blood supply in the dermal papilla. A longer, quiescent period **(telogen)** then takes place. The hair (now a **club hair**) separates from the hair bulb matrix but remains in the follicle. The hair bulb matrix later becomes active, contacts the dermal papilla and begins to grow a new hair. The new, growing hair pushes out the old club hair **(shedding)**. Hairs are shed periodically, mostly in the spring, but, in some breeds, shedding may occur throughout the year.

Alopecia (loss of hair), reddening and crusting of the skin, and generalized demodectic mange are all accompanied by pruritis (itching) and may be manifestations of systemic disease.

Figure 1

Figure 2

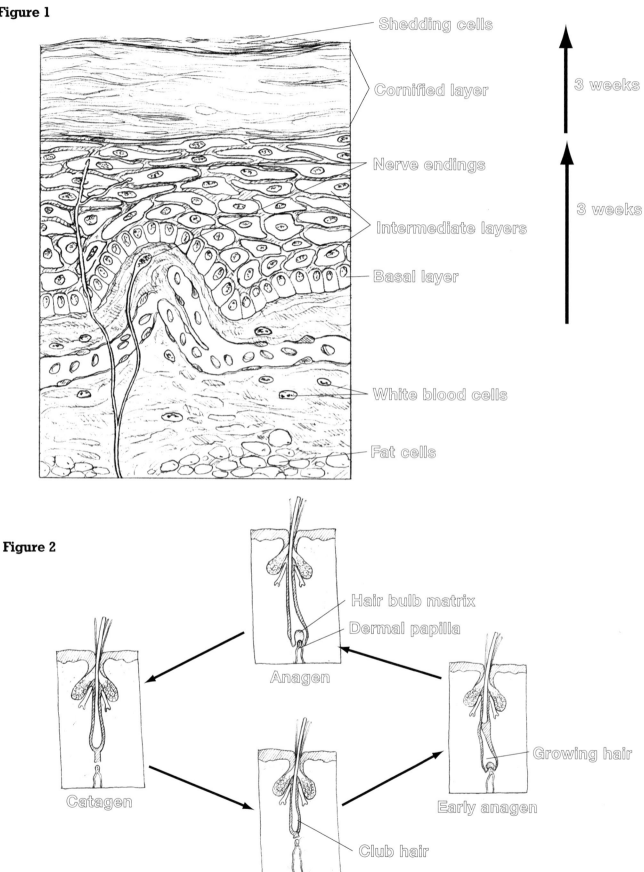

Shedding cells

Cornified layer

3 weeks

Nerve endings

3 weeks

Intermediate layers

Basal layer

White blood cells

Fat cells

Hair bulb matrix

Dermal papilla

Anagen

Growing hair

Catagen

Early anagen

Club hair

Telogen

Types of Hair Coats

PLATE 6

Cats hairs vary from straight, tapered guard hairs to wool hairs of the undercoat and the soft vellus hairs of kittens, Vellus hairs are the kitten's only hairs in the first few weeks after birth. Then the guard hairs and wool hairs emerge from their follicles.

Adult cats of most breeds possess a **double coat** consisting of a primary (guard) hair and two types of secondary (fur or wool) hairs: 1. Awn hairs have a swelling just below the tip. 2. Down hairs are the thinnest hairs and are crimped or wavy. All of the hairs have a medulla. Cats have compound hair follicles - a primary hair and a few secondary hairs emerge through one opening in the skin. Guard hairs form a protective, outer **cover coat**; the two finer secondary hairs make up the **undercoat**. Secondary hairs form the supporting undercoat, providing an insulating, water-resistant barrier. Longer guard hairs form the feathering on limbs and the plumes on tails. Secondary hairs outnumber the primary hairs in greater numbers ventrally (24:1) than dorsally (10:1).

The typical double coat occurs in the **longhair (A)** and **shorthair (B)** breeds and in most crossbred cats. A curly coat in the **Rex breeds (C)** and the wire coat of the **Wirehair American breeds (D)** are mutant hair coats.

The skin of a **hairless (E)** cat contains a few stunted hairs. Larger hairs appear on the head (crest), tail (plume), manus and pes (socks). The skin of these cats contains well-developed sweat glands.

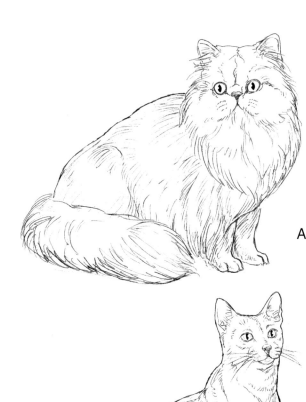

A. Longhair (Persian)

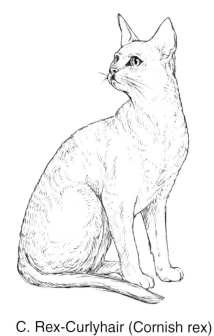

C. Rex-Curlyhair (Cornish rex)

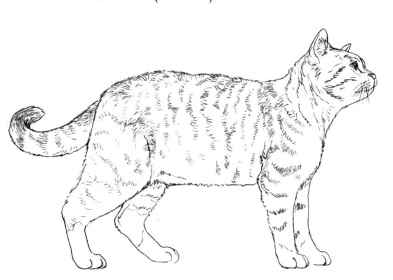

B. Shorthair (Havana)

D. Wirehair (Tabby)

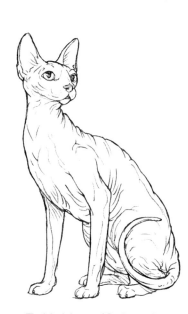

E. Hairless (Sphynx)

Organs of Movement:
Bones, Joints, and Muscles

Skeleton

PLATE 7

A cat will have between 230 and 245 bones (24 more than people when full grown) and will have fewer bones as they get older because of bones fusing together.

Underline the name of each bone with a different color and use the same color on the labeled bone.

AXIAL SKELETON

1. Skull
2. Mandible
3. Hyoid apparatus
4. Vertebral column
5. Ribs
6. Costal cartilages
   (several small bones)
7. Sternum

APPENDICULAR SKELETON

FORELIMB

8. Clavicle
9. Scapula
10. Humerus
11. Radius
12. Ulna
13. Carpal bones (7)
14. Metacarpal bones (5)
15. Palmar sesamoid bones (9)
    (Singular = phalanx)
16. Proximal phalanges (5)
17. Middle phalanges (4)
18. Claw
19. Distal phalanges (5)

HINDLIMB

20. Ilium
21. Pubis
22. Ischium ⎱ Fused to form
23. Femur ⎰ the hip bone
     (os coxae)
24. Patella
25. Fabellae (3)
26. Tibia
27. Fibula
28. Tarsal bones (7)
29. Metatarsal bones (5)
30. Penile bone (baculum)

Hindlimb digital bones are named the same as those of the forelimb.
A dewclaw (1st digit) is rarely present.

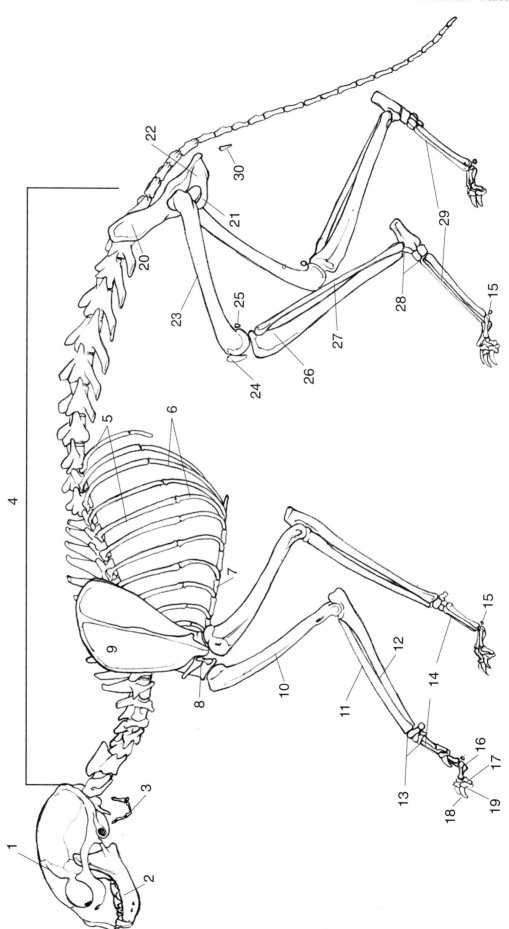

Vertebral (Spinal) Column

PLATE 8

Figure 1. Regions of the vertebral (spinal) column.

Color in the vertebral regions and the number of vertebrae in each region:
7 cervical, 13 thoracic, 7 lumbar, 3 sacral (fused by 1 1/2 years to form the **sacrum**) and **18-20 caudal (coccygeal) vertebrae**.
Next to the wide variation in the number of caudal vertebrae, the most common variation is 6 lumbar vertebrae.
The <u>vertebral formula</u> of the cat is written $C_7 \, T_{13} \, L_7 \, S_3 \, Ca_{18-20}$

Figure 2. Vertebrae are irregular bones of various shapes.

Identify and color the parts of vertebrae from different regions:
1. **Transverse processes** (**Wings** on the atlas and sacrum)
2. **Dens** of the axis (Held down by the transverse ligament of the atlas)
3. **Transverse foramen** (On all cervical vertebrae except the seventh)
4. **Lateral vertebral foramen**
5. **Vertebral foramen** (Combined vertebral foramina form the <u>vertebral canal</u> which contains and protects the spinal cord and its coverings.)
6. **Body**
7. **Arch**
8. **Spinous process**
9. **Articular processes**
10. **Left articular surface of sacrum**. (Articulates with ilium)
11. **Dorsal sacral foramina**

Except for articulations of the atlas with the skull (atlanto-occipital joint) and with the axis (atlanto-axial joint - a pivot joint), the bodies of vertebrae are joined by **intervertebral disks** of fibrous cartilage. Movements of vertebral joints (except the atlanto-axial joint) are dorsal, ventral and lateral flexion. There is also limited rotation.

Spinal nerves come out through foramina formed between arches of adjacent vertebrae. On each side, a <u>vertebral artery</u> runs through foramina in the transverse processes of cervical vertebrae six through one (the atlas) and through the lateral vertebral foramen of the atlas to contribute to the blood supply to the brain.

Figure 1

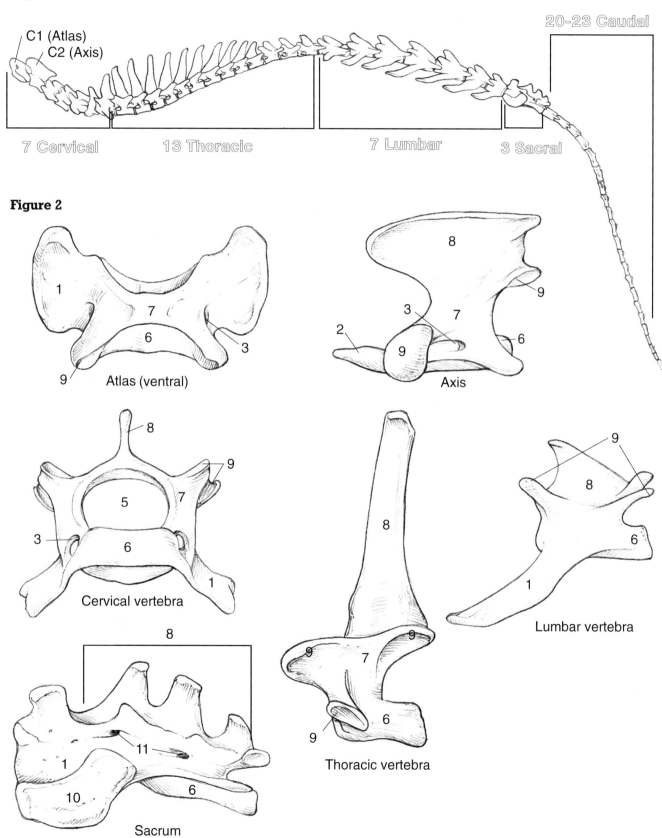

C1 (Atlas)
C2 (Axis)

20-23 Caudal

7 Cervical   13 Thoracic   7 Lumbar   3 Sacral

Figure 2

Atlas (ventral)

Axis

Cervical vertebra

Thoracic vertebra

Lumbar vertebra

Sacrum

Ribs and Sternum

PLATE 9

The cat has 13 pairs (rarely 12 or 14 pairs) of **ribs** (L., *costa* = rib), each rib consisting of a bony part joined to a **costal cartilage** at a **costochondral junction** (Greek, *chondros* = cartilage). The costal cartilages of the first nine pairs of ribs articulate with the **sternum** at **chondrosternal junctions**; the last four pairs are asternal ribs. Since their cartilages do not attach to adjacent costal cartilages, the **13th ribs** are called floating ribs. Fused costal cartilages form the **costal arch**. Most of the bony ribs, the **costal arch** and the sternum can be palpated (felt) from the exterior.

Figure 1. Left lateral view of ribs, sternum and thoracic vertebrae.

The **head** of each rib 1 through 10 or 11 articulates with the bodies of adjacent vertebrae and the intervertebral disc between them. The head of the **first rib** articulates with the bodies of the **7th cervical (C7)** and **1st thoracic (T1) vertebrae**. Ribs 11 or 12 through 13 articulate only with thoracic vertebrae of the same number. The **tubercle** on ribs 1 through 10 or 11 articulates with the transverse process of the thoracic vertebra of the same number. On the caudal ribs of the series, the **neck** of the rib becomes shorter as the tubercle approaches the head and eventually fuses with it.

Figure 2. Ventral view of ribs and sternum.

The **sternum** consists of eight elongated, bony **sternebrae** joined by **intersternal cartilages**. The first sternebra is called the **manubrium**; the eighth sternebra, the **xiphoid process**. A thin, flat plate, the **xiphoid cartilage**, extends caudad from the xiphoid process.

Figure 1

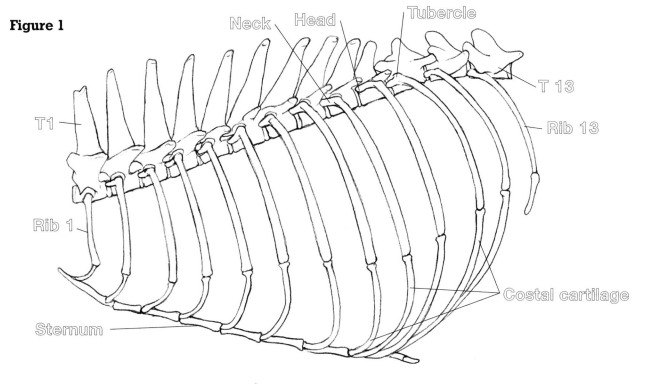

Figure 2

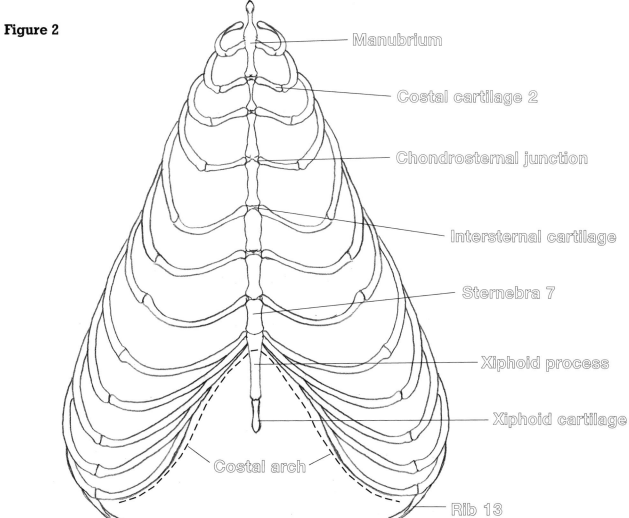

Bones of the Shoulder, Arm and Forearm

PLATE 10

Figure 1. Lateral and medial views of the left scapula, humerus, radius and ulna. Underline the names and color the parts of the bones different colors.

1. Supraspinous fossa
2. Spine
3. Acromion
   a. Hamate process
   b. Suprahamate process
4. Infraspinous fossa
5. Supraglenoid tubercle
6. Coracoid process
7. Serrated face
8. Subscapular fossa
9. Glenoid cavity
10. Greater tubercle
11. Intertubercular groove
12. Lesser tubercle
13. Head
14. Deltoid tuberosity
15. Brachial groove
16. Teres major tuberosity
17. Lateral epicondyle
18. Supracondylar foramen
19. Medial epicondyle
20. Articular circumference
21. Neck
22. Radial tuberosity
23. Olecranon tuber
24. Carpal articular surface
25. Lateral styloid process – ulna
26. Medial styloid process – radius

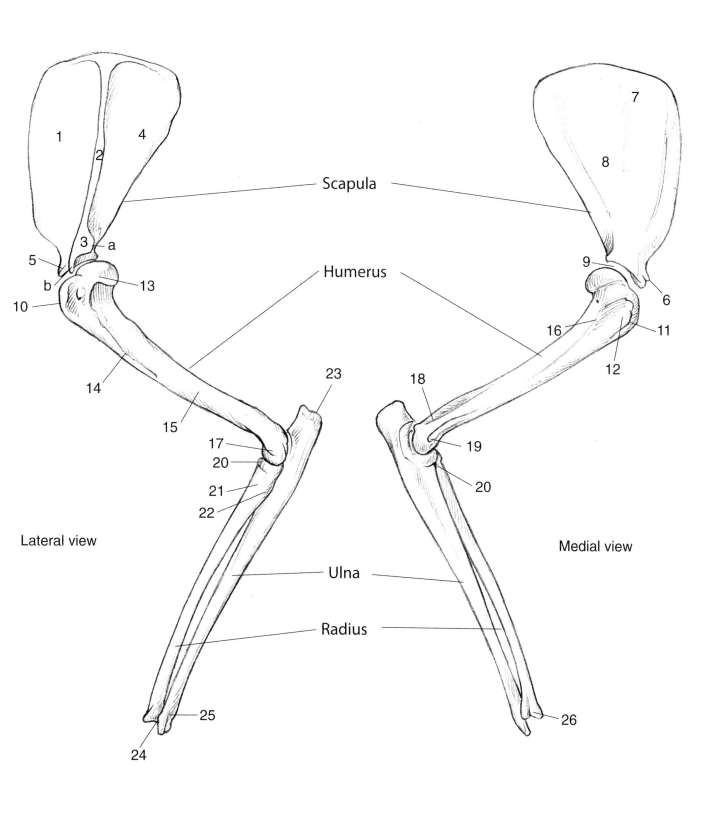

Scapula

Humerus

Lateral view

Medial view

Ulna

Radius

Carpal, Metacarpal and Digital Bones

PLATE 11

Dorsal view of the bones of the left carpus, metacarpus and forefoot (forepaw) with the bones slightly disarticulated.

Using a different color for each of the four groups below, underline the names of the bones in the group. Use the same colors for the labeled bones on the plate.

Carpal bones:
1. **Radial carpal bone**
2. **Ulnar carpal bone**
3. **Accessory carpal bone**
4. **First carpal bone**
5. **Second carpal bone**
6. **Third carpal bone**
7. **Fourth carpal bone**

Metacarpal bones:
8. **First metacarpal bone**
9. **Second metacarpal bone**
10. **Third metacarpal bone**
11. **Fourth metacarpal bone**
12. **Fifth metacarpal bone**

Sesamoid bones:
13. **Sesamoid bone** in the tendon of the long abductor of the pollex (thumb).
14. **Metacarpophalangeal sesamoid bones**
Sesamoid bones are attached to or embedded in tendons of muscles. A sesamoid bone protects a tendon where it moves against a joint surface, acting as a pulley to change the tendon's direction of pull.

Digital bones (phalanges; singular, phalanx):
15. **Proximal phalanges - I, II, III, IV, V**
16. **Middle phalanges - II, III, IV, V**
17. **Distal phalanges - I, II, III, IV, V**

On each distal phalanx note the **ungual crest** and **ungual process** which is enclosed by the claw.

Dorsal view

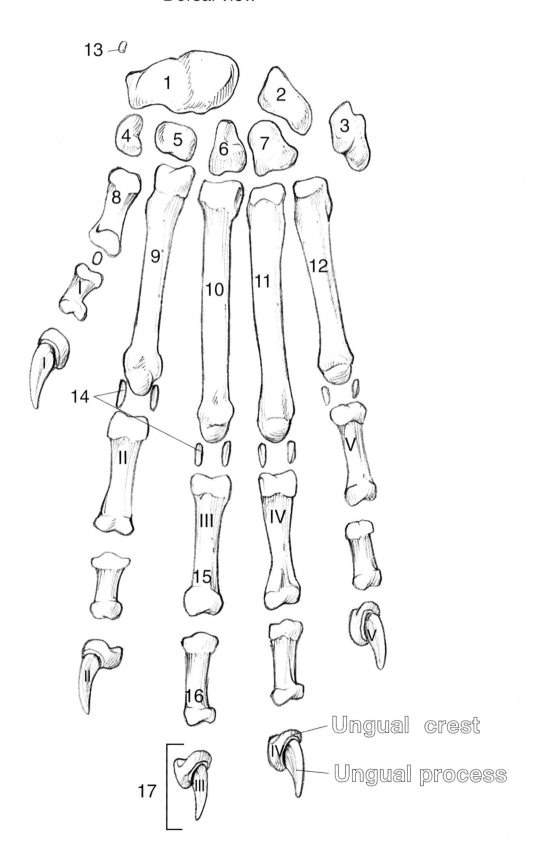

13

1

2

3

4   5   6   7

8

9   10   11   12

I

I

14

II

III   IV

V

V

15

II

III   IV

V

16

Ungual crest

IV

17   III

Ungual process

Structure of Joints

PLATE 12

Figure 1. <u>Fibrous joints</u> - Immovable; united by fibrous tissue; ossify with age.
    Suture - Most joints of the skull.
    Syndesmosis - Between the shafts of some long bones.

Figure 2. <u>Cartilaginous joints</u> - Limited movement; midline.
    Symphysis - Fibrocartilage. Pelvic symphysis ossifies with age. Intervertebral discs do not normally ossify.
    Growth plate (physis) (arrows) - Hyaline cartilage grows and calcifies, providing a scaffold upon which bone is deposited. This process causes a bone to grow in length. At maturity the physis is completely ossified. Growth plate fractures occur in young cats.

Figure 3. <u>Synovial joint</u> - Drawn here in longitudinal section. Synovial (<u>diarthrodial</u>) joints are movable.

    Parts of a typical synovial joint. Color the parts indicated.
    Articular cartilages - Smooth, glassy <u>hyaline cartilage</u>.
    Synovial membrane - Produces lubricating <u>synovial fluid</u> ("joint oil").
    Fibrous joint capsule
    Collateral ligaments - Extra-articular.
    <u>Intra-articular ligaments</u> in the femorotibial joint of the <u>stifle</u> are <u>not</u> within the synovial cavity. In this joint, <u>menisci of fibrocartilage</u> are placed between the articulating bones.

Synovial joints are classified also on the basis of the shape of articular surfaces and type of motion:
    <u>Hinge joint</u> (<u>ginglymus</u>) - <u>Flexion</u> decreases the angle between the bones in a joint; <u>extension</u> increases the angle: elbow joint.
    <u>Sliding joint</u> (<u>plane joint</u>): intercarpal joints - between carpal bones.
    <u>Ball-and-socket joint</u> (<u>spheroidal joint</u>): hip joint.
    <u>Pivot joint</u> (<u>trochoid joint</u>): atlanto-axial joint.
    <u>Ellipsoid joint</u> - Biaxial movement: antebrachiocarpal joint.
    <u>Saddle joints</u>: the cat's interphalangeal joints.
The initial swelling of an injured joint is due to increased production of synovial fluid. Analysis of the viscosity (thickness) of the synovial fluid and cells that it contains is used to diagnose certain joint diseases.

Figure 1. Fibrous joints

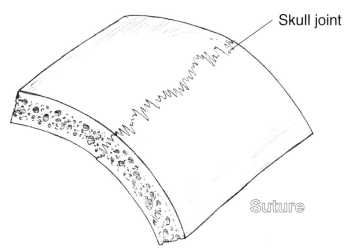

Skull joint

Suture

Figure 2. Cartilaginous joints

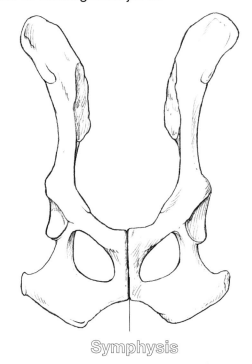

Symphysis

Syndesmosis

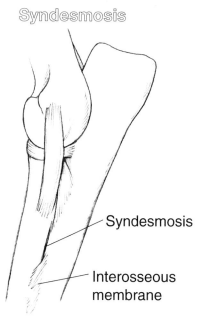

Syndesmosis

Interosseous membrane

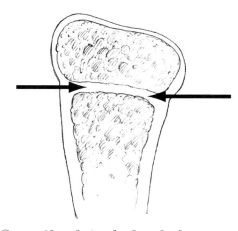

Growth plate (physis)

Figure 3. Synovial joint

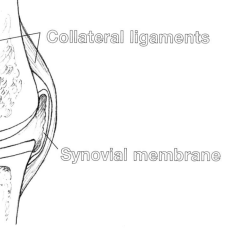

Collateral ligaments

Articular cartilage

Fibrous joint capsule

Synovial membrane

Joints of the Forelimb

PLATE 13

On the plate, color the names and draw a colored line through the joints indicated.

Shoulder (humeral) joint - Glenoid cavity of scapula with head of humerus. Surrounding muscles act as ligaments. This is a ball-and-socket joint but main movements are flexion and extension.

Elbow (cubital) joint - Condyle of humerus with capitular fovea of radius and trochlear notch of ulna. It includes the proximal radioulnar joint between the articular circumference of the radius and the radial notch of the ulna. The joint capsule extends a pouch into the olecranon fossa. The joint is a ginglymus.

Interosseous ligament of the forearm (antebrachium) - Between apposed rough areas on the shafts of the radius and ulna.

Distal radioulnar joint - Between radius and ulna distally. Contains an extension of the antebrachiocarpal joint capsule. Allows some rotation.

Carpal joints - Together act as a ginglymus.
    Antebrachiocarpal joint - Between distal ends of radius and ulna and proximal row of carpal bones. Major joint of the carpus.
    Middle carpal joint - Between proximal row and distal row of carpal bones.
    Carpometacarpal joint - Between distal row of carpal bones and proximal ends (bases) of metacarpal bones.
    Intercarpal joints - Between individual carpal bones.
    Several small ligaments between adjacent bones, short radial carpal ligaments and a short ulnar carpal ligament bind the carpal joints. The palmar carpal fibrocartilage attaches to all of the carpal bones except the accessory carpal and forms the deep smooth surface of the carpal canal. The fibrous flexor retinaculum and accessory carpal bone complete the formation of the canal, enclosing digital flexor tendons, blood vessels and nerves.

Intermetacarpal joints - Between proximal ends of adjacent metacarpal bones.

Metacarpophalangeal joints - Between distal ends of metacarpal bones and proximal ends of proximal phalanges. Various sesamoidean ligaments stabilize the pair of palmar sesamoid bones embedded in the tendon of the interosseous muscle at each of the four main joints.

Proximal interphalangeal joints - Between proximal and middle phalanges.

Distal interphalangeal joints - Between middle and distal phalanges. Collateral ligaments bind the interphalangeal joints. A **dorsal elastic ligament** extends from the middle phalanx to the ungual crest of the distal phalanx.

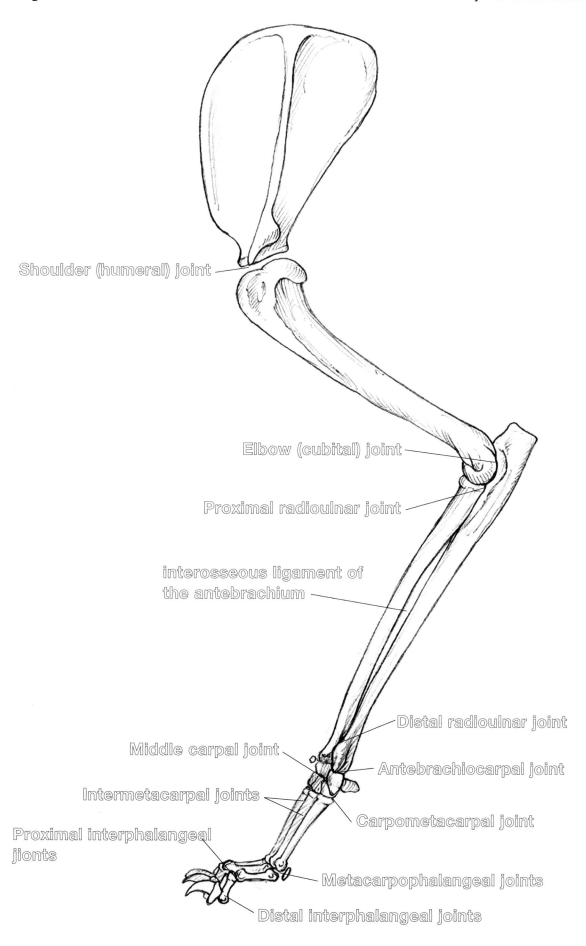

Shoulder (humeral) joint

Elbow (cubital) joint

Proximal radioulnar joint

interosseous ligament of
the antebrachium

Distal radioulnar joint

Middle carpal joint

Antebrachiocarpal joint

Intermetacarpal joints

Carpometacarpal joint

Proximal interphalangeal
jionts

Metacarpophalangeal joints

Distal interphalangeal joints

Fascia

PLATE 14

When removing the skin from an animal, the lacy subcutis of loose connective tissue is seen as it is pulled away from the superficial fascia. The latter varies from loose to dense connective tissue that envelops the body and contains certain cutaneous muscles of the head, neck and trunk. The largest of these is the cutaneus trunci m. (cutaneous muscle of the trunk) that covers a large part of the thorax and abdomen. Deep to the superficial fascia, thick, white deep fascia of heavier dense connective tissue encloses muscles and sends partitions called septa between muscles and some muscle parts. Before the limits of many muscles can be seen clearly, fascia has to be cleaned, that is, removed. Fascia covers joints and blends with ligaments, tendons and tendon sheaths.

Color the names of the region of fascia and the cutaneous muscles. Color the cutaneous muscles.

CUTANEOUS MUSCLES

Platysma muscle

Sphincter muscles of the neck

Cutaneous muscle of the trunk (m. cutaneus trunci)

MAJOR REGIONS OF FASCIA

Fascia of the head

Cervical fascia

Omobrachial fascia

Spinotransverse fascia
(deep to the shoulder)

Thoracolumbar fascia

Abdominal fascia

Gluteal fascia

Tail fascia

Lateral femoral fascia (Fascia lata)

Medial femoral fascia
(on medial aspect of the thigh)

Crural fascia

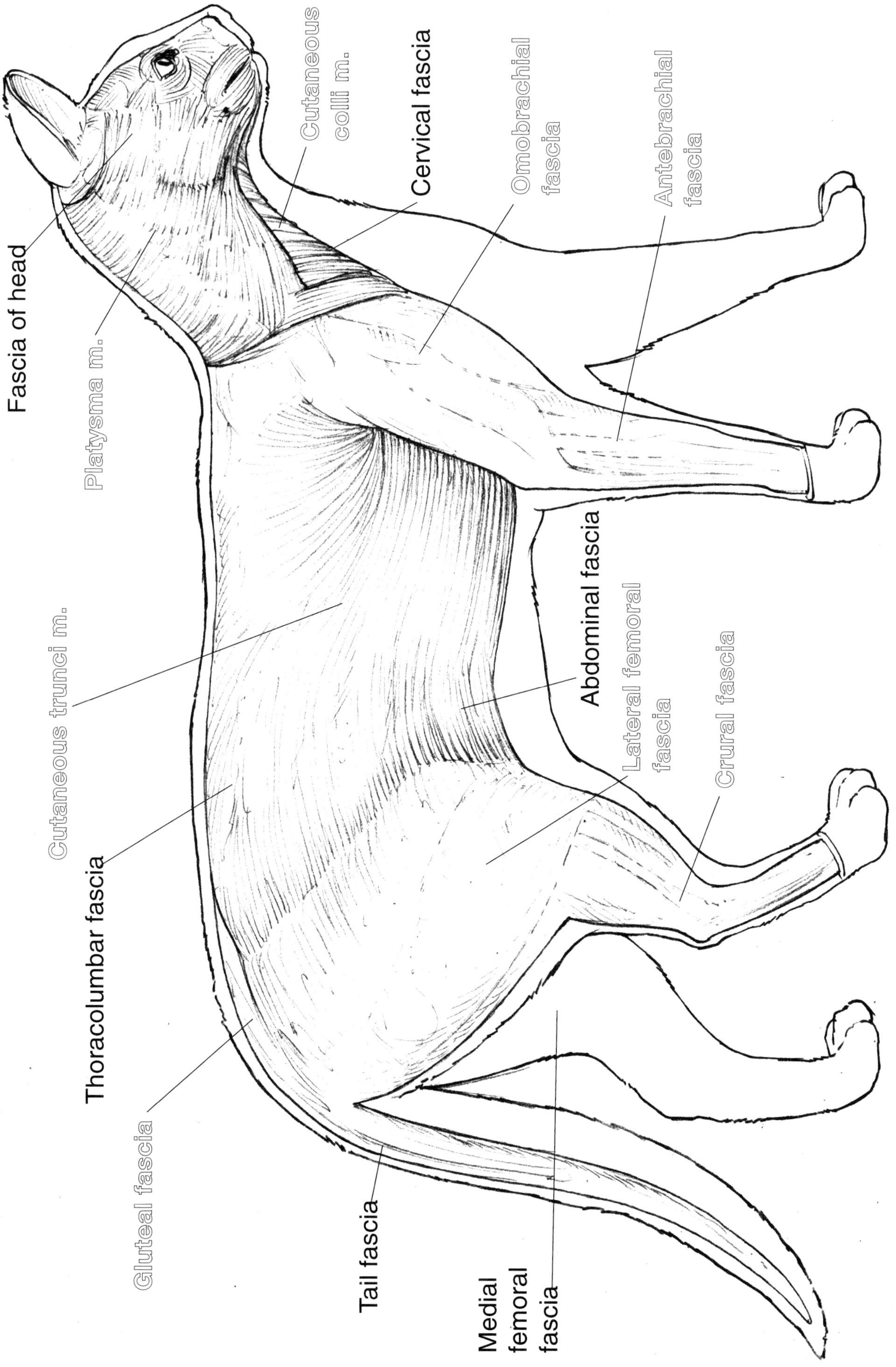

Fascia of head

Platysma m.

Cutaneous colli m.

Cervical fascia

Omobrachial fascia

Antebrachial fascia

Cutaneous trunci m.

Abdominal fascia

Lateral femoral fascia

Crural fascia

Thoracolumbar fascia

Gluteal fascia

Tail fascia

Medial femoral fascia

Superficial Muscles

PLATE 15

Left lateral view of the superficial muscles after removal of most of the fascia and the cutaneous muscles.

Underline names and color the muscles indicated on the drawing. m. = muscle. The cleidocervical m. and cleidobrachial m. are parts of the brachiocephalic m.

1. Nasolabial levator m.
2. Orbicular ocular m.
3. Temporal m.
4. Frontal m.
5. Oral orbicular m.
6. Parotidoauricular muscle
7. Masseter m.
8. Digastric m.
9. Sternohyoid m.
10. Sternocephalic m.
11. Cleidocervical m.
12. Trapezius m.
13. Omotransverse m.
14. Clavicular tendon in brachiocephalic m.

15. Cleidobrachial m.
16. Deltoid m. (2 parts)
17. Brachioradialis m.
18. Brachial triceps m.
19. Deep pectoral m
20. Latissimus dorsi m.
21. External abdominal oblique m.
22. Gastrocnemius m.
23. Sacrocaudal mm.
24. Superficial and middle gluteal mm.
25. Sartorial m.
26. Tensor m. of fascia lata
27. Femoral biceps m.
28. Semitendinous m.

Skeletal muscle is voluntary, i. e., under control of the will. Under a microscope, its fibers (cells) are striated (striped across) due to the arrangement of molecules within the fibers. The fibers of cardiac (heart) muscle are also striated, but the beating is involuntary. The third muscle type, smooth muscle, is nonstriated, and its contractions are involuntary. Smooth muscle occurs in blood vessels, intestines, bladder and uterus. Muscles function in locomotion, breathing, circulation, digestion and reproduction. Muscles are also responsible for facial expression, hair raising, tail movement and vocalization.

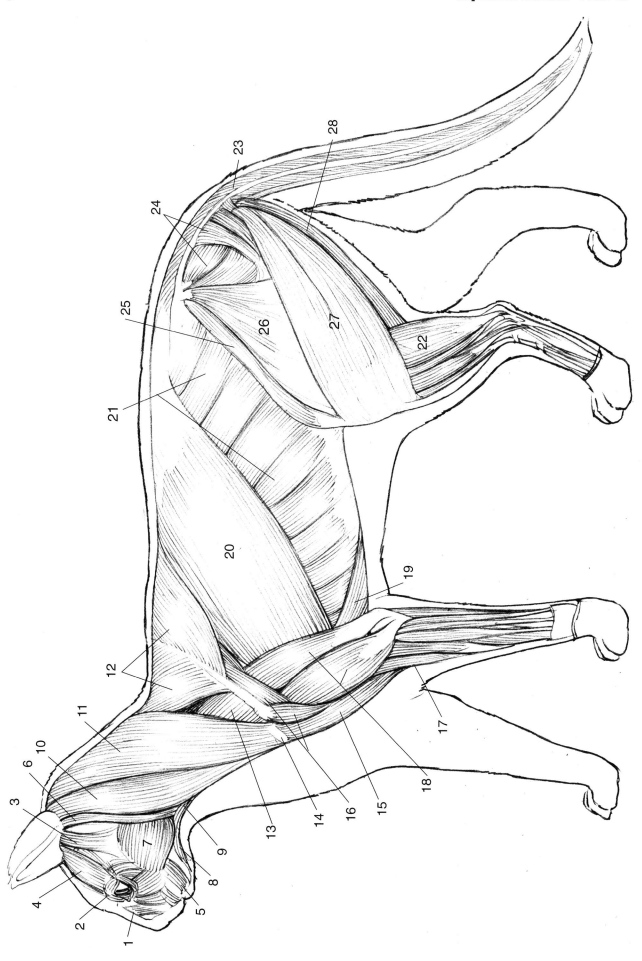

Deep Muscles

PLATE 16

Figure 1. Left lateral view of deeper muscles of trunk and proximal parts of the limbs. m. = muscle
Figure 2. Ventral view of muscles of shoulders and chest.

Underline the names below and color the muscles indicated on the plate.

1. Long head m.
2. Complexus m.
3. Hyoglossus m.
4. Genohyoid m.
5. Esophagus
6. Sternohyoid m.
7. Sternothyroid m.
8. Infraspinate m.
9. Supraspinate m.
10. Brachial triceps m. (intermediate portion)
11. Brachial m.
12. Anconeous m.
13. Supinator m.
14. Long extensor of pollex m.

15. Ventral cranial serrated m.
16. Dorsal spinal and semispinal m.
17. Longest thoracic and lumbar m.
18. Lumbar iliocostal m.
19. Transversospinal m.
20. Semispinalis head m
21. Long abductor pollex m.
22. Deep head of deep digital flexor m.
23. Capsular m
24. Medial vast m.
25. Femoral adductor m.
26. Interosseus ligament
27. Long flexor hallux m.

Extensor muscles draw two members of a joint away from each other. The action is called <u>extension</u>.
<u>Flexor muscles</u> draw two members of a joint together. The action is called flexion.

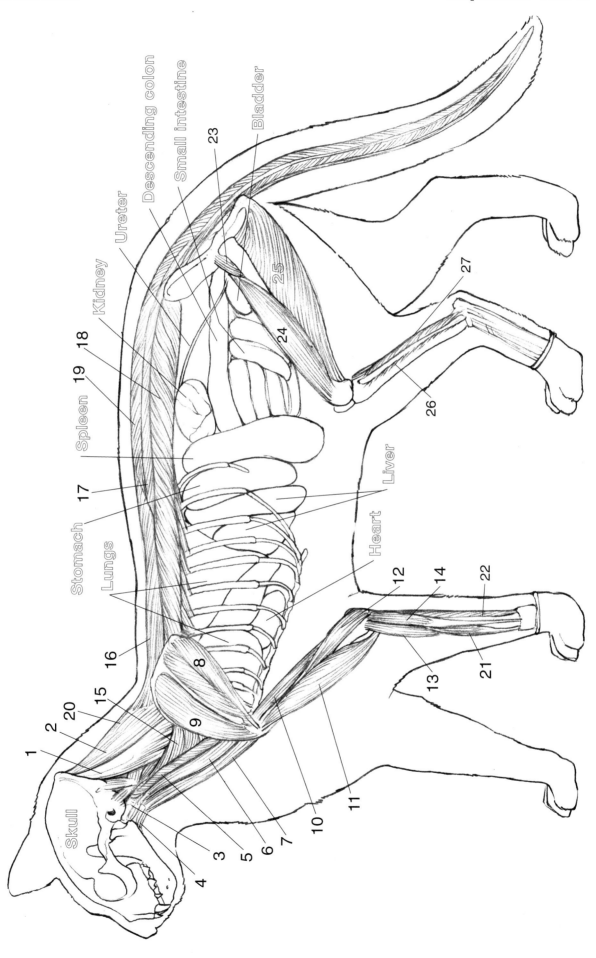

Skull

Stomach

Lungs

Spleen

Kidney

Ureter

Descending colon

Small intestine

Bladder

Heart

Liver

1
2
20
15
17
19
18
16
9
8
5
3
4
6
7
10
11
13
21
22
14
12
26
27
25
24
23

Deep Shoulder and Arm Muscles

PLATE 17

Figure 1. Lateral view of left shoulder and arm muscles. m. = muscle
Figure 2. Medial view of left shoulder and arm muscles. The limb is cut away from the trunk.

As you color the muscles indicated, try to determine their actions from their positions and the joints they cross. See the actions (results of muscular contractions) summarized in the paragraph below.

1. **Infraspinatus m.**
2. **Teres major m.**
3. **Supraspinatus m.**
4. **Spinous part of deltoid m.**
5. **Acromial part of deltoid m.**
6a. **Long head of biceps m.**
6b. **Lateral head of triceps m.**
6c. **Medial head of triceps m.**
6d. **Acessory head of triceps m.**
7. **Brachialis m.**

8. **Brachial biceps m.**
9. **Brachioradial m.**
10. **Subscapular m.**
11. **Coracobrachial m.**
12. **Radial carpal extensor m.**
13. **Deep digital flexor m.**
14. **Pronator teres m.**
15. **Radial carpal flexor m.**
16. **Superficial digital flexor m.**

The forelimb is elevated by the **rhomboid m. pectoral, supraspinate, coracobrachial** and **subscapular muscles** extend the shoulder joint; the **teres muscles** flex it and rotate the shoulder inward. The **infraspinate m.** rotates the shoulder outward and, with the **supraspinate m.,** serves as the lateral collateral ligament of the shoulder joint. The main extensor of the shoulder, the **brachial triceps m.,** is aided by the **anconeal m.** The **brachial biceps** and **brachial muscles** flex the elbow joint.

Figure 2

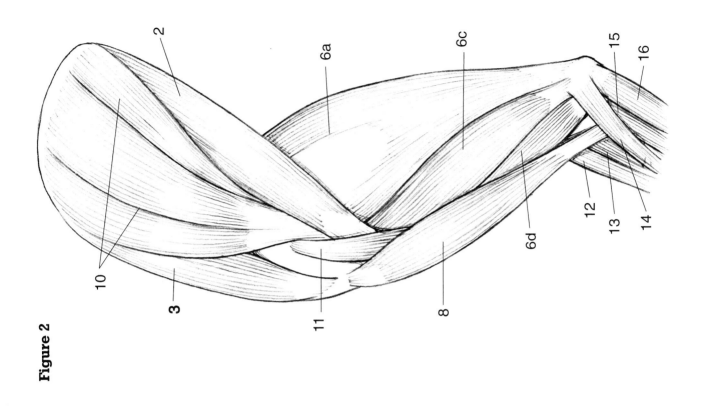

Figure 1

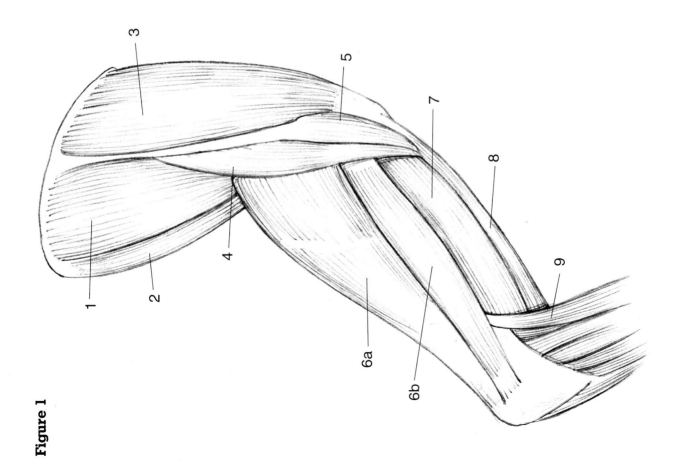

Forearm and Forefoot Muscles

PLATE 18

Dissections of left forearm and forefoot (forepaw) muscles and tendons attaching to the carpal bones, metacarpal bones and phalanges. m. = muscle

Underline the names below and color the muscles indicated on the plate.

1. Biceps
2. Triceps
3. Brachioradialis
4. Extensor carpi radialis
5. Common digital extensor
6. Long abductor m. of first digit
7. Carpal retinaculum
8. Tendons of the digital extensors
9. Lateral digital extensor

10. Lumbricals
11. Lateral digital extensor
12. Extensor carpi ulnaris
13. Flexor carpi ulnaris
14. Pronator teres
15. Superficial digital flexor
16. Flexor carpi radialis
17. Deep digital flexor
18. Abductor pollicis longus

An underlined muscle pulls a limb part away from the limb axis or a limb away from the trunk. The action is called abduction. The opposite term is adduction, the movement of a limb toward the trunk.

Pronator muscles rotate the forearm so that the palmar surface of the forepaw is directed laterad and thus to the ground (pronation). A **supinator muscle** (not seen here) aided by the brachioradial m. acts to rotate the forearm so that the palmar surface of the paw is directed medially. This action is greater in the cat than in the dog.

Notice that the tendons of the deep digital flexor m. perforate the tendons of the superficial digital flexor m. as they extend to their attachments on the digits.

Lateral view

Medial view

Forelimb Nerves

PLATE 19

Nerves supplying the forelimb muscles and sensation to the forelimb originate from the **brachial plexus**, a network formed by the ventral branches of the last three cervical and first one or two thoracic spinal nerves coming from the cervical swelling of the spinal cord.

The plate is a medial view of the left forelimb skeleton with the courses of the main forelimb nerves drawn roughly upon it.

Underline the names and trace the course of each nerve indicated by its matching number in a different color. n. = nerve

1. **Subscapular n.** - supplies subscapular muscle

2. **Suprascapular n.** - around neck of scapula to supply supraspinate and infraspinate muscles

3. **Axillary n.** - to deltoid, major teres, minor teres and subscapular muscles

4. **Radial n.** - to brachial triceps, radial carpal extensor, lateral ulnar supinator, brachioradialis, common and lateral digital extensors

5. **Musculocutaneous n.** - to brachial biceps, coracobrachialis and brachial

6. **Median n.** - supplies radial carpal flexor, pronator, superficial digital flexor, deep digital flexor muscles; sensory to caudal forearm and palmar paw skin over digits 2,3,4

7. **Ulnar n.** - supplies ulnar carpal flexor and deep digital flexor muscles

8. **Deep branch of radial n.** - to all extensor muscles of the carpus and digits

9. **Medial cutaneous antebrachial n.** – sensory to medial forearm skin

10. **Cranial cutaneous antebrachial n.** - sensory to cranial forearm skin

11. **Superficial branch of radial n.** - sensory to dorsal forearm and paw

12. **Caudal cutaneous antebrachial n.** - sensory to caudal forearm

13. **Dorsal branch of ulnar n.** - sensory to dorsal skin of digit 5

14. **Palmar branch of ulnar n.** - to paw muscles; sensory to skin over digit 5

Other nerves from the brachial plexus supply the pectoral, brachiocephalic, ventral serrated, cutaneous trunk and widest dorsal (latissimus dorsi) muscles as well as the diaphragm via the phrenic nerve.

Injury to the radial nerve causes paralysis of the muscles it supplies. If it is damaged at the proximal end of the humerus, the forelimb cannot give support to the body because the brachial triceps cannot extend the elbow. Damage to the radial nerve in the region of the elbow results in lack of extension of the carpus and digits, and the cat supports its weight on the dorsal surface of the forefoot.

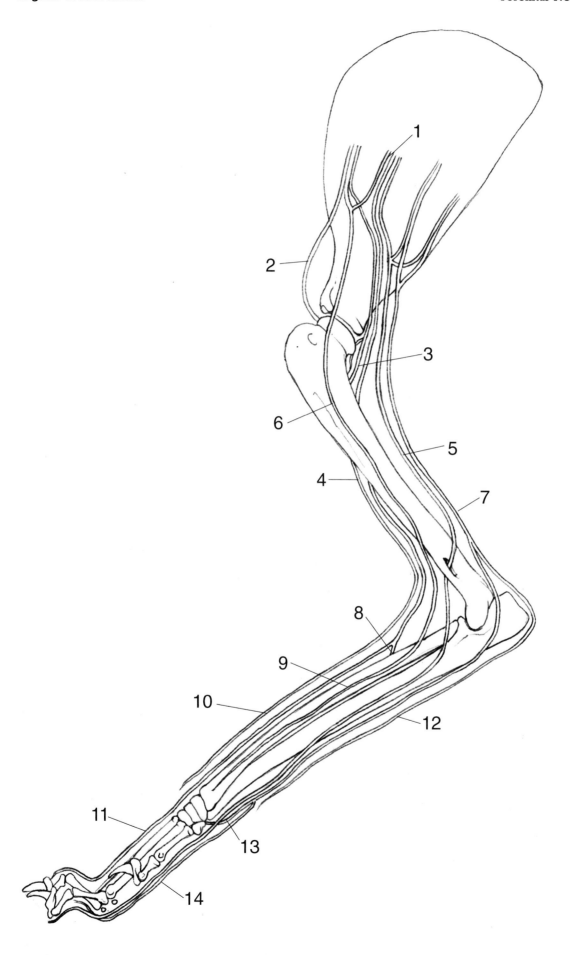

Forelimb Blood Vessels

PLATE 20

In these drawings, the courses of the vessels are related roughly to the skeleton of the right forelimb. Diameters of some of the smaller vessels are larger than normal to permit coloring.

Color the names on the plate and underline the names below on the plate. Color the vessels indicated, using red for arteries and blue for veins.

1. **Thoracodorsal a. & v.**
2. **Caudal circumflex humeral a.**
3. **Cranial circumflex humeral a.**
4. **Deep brachial a. & v.**
5. **Superficial brachial a.**
6. **Collateral ulnar a. & v.**
7. **Cranial superficial antebrachial a.**
8. **Cranial interosseous a.**

Blood reaches the forefoot primarily through the **axillary, brachial** and **median aa.** Secondary blood supplies are provided by the **common interosseous, caudal interosseous** and **radial aa.** and the cranial **superficial antebrachial a.** Arteries to the metacarpus and digits arise from the **superficial** and **deep palmar arches, cranial superficial antebrachial a.** and **dorsal carpal rete** (Latin, network).

Notice that most veins are satellites of arteries, but there are some differences between the venous drainage of the forelimb and its arterial supply. In addition to satellite veins, blood is drained from the forelimb by the **accessory cephalic, cephalic, median cubital** and **omobrachial vv.** The **cephalic** and **omobrachial vv.** carry blood to the external jugular v. The **cranial superficial antebrachial a.** and its **medial branch** lie one on either side of the cephalic vein. Veins from the metacarpus and digits return blood to the **proximal** and **distal palmar venous arches** and the **accessory cephalic v.**

Veins differ from arteries in that they:
  a. contain a larger volume of blood.
  b. have thinner walls.
  c. usually have valves, they direct blood to heart.

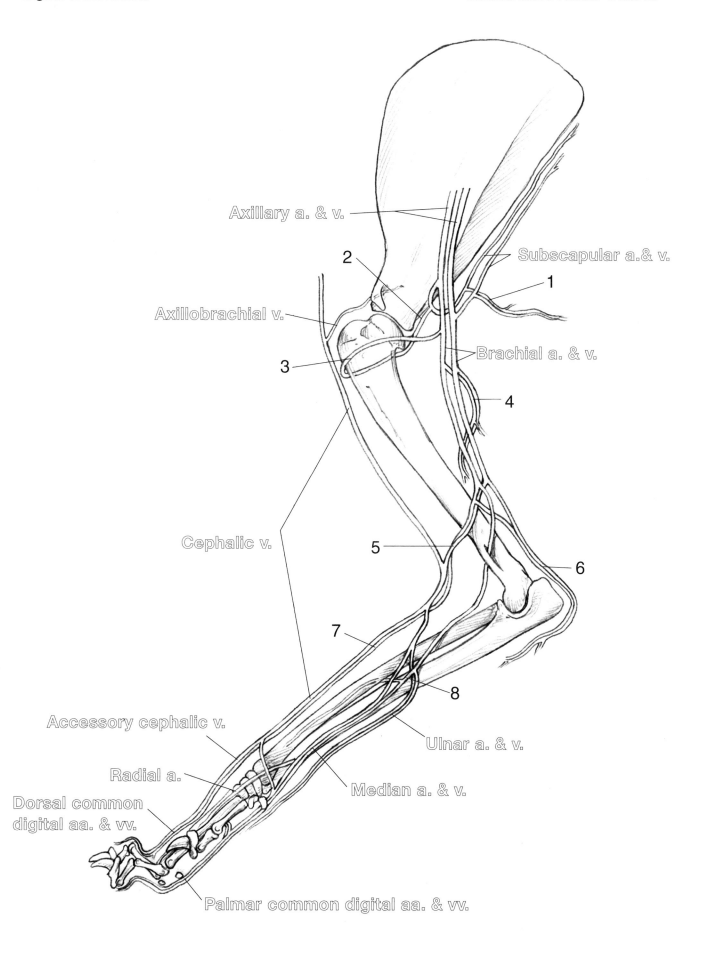

Axillary a. & v.

Subscapular a.& v.

2

1

Axillobrachial v.

3

Brachial a. & v.

4

Cephalic v.

5

6

7

8

Accessory cephalic v.

Ulnar a. & v.

Radial a.

Dorsal common
digital aa. & vv.

Median a. & v.

Palmar common digital aa. & vv.

Forepaw

PLATE 21

The terms, foot and paw, have been used interchangeably. On Plate 1, notice that the forefoot or forepaw (L., *manus*, hand) consists of the carpus, metacarpus and digits; the hindfoot or hindpaw (L. *pes*, foot) consists of the tarsus, metatarsus and digits. Only the distal parts of the metacarpus or metatarsus and the digits are considered to be the paw. The pastern includes the metacarpus or metatarsus.

Underline the numbered names below and color the structures indicated

Figure 1.
   a. Palmar view of left forefoot. The **carpal pad** (stopper pad) touches the ground only when a rapidly running cat corners.
   b. Plantar view of the left hindfoot. There is no pad over the tarsus.

Figure 2.
   a. Superficial palmar dissection of left forefoot with footpads intact.
   b. Deeper palmar dissection of left forefoot.

Figure 1

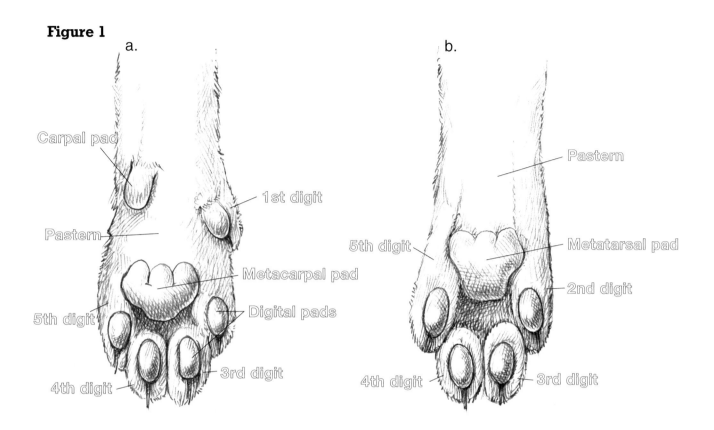

a.

Carpal pad

Pastern

5th digit

4th digit

1st digit

Metacarpal pad

Digital pads

3rd digit

b.

Pastern

Metatarsal pad

5th digit

2nd digit

4th digit

3rd digit

Figure 2

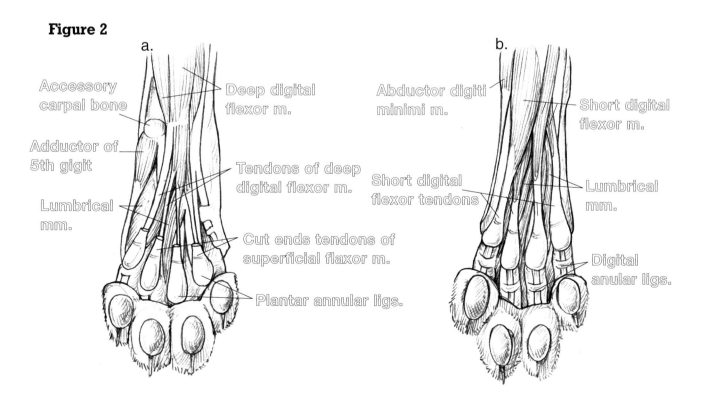

a.

Accessory
carpal bone

Adductor of
5th gigit

Lumbrical
mm.

Deep digital
flexor m.

Tendons of deep
digital flexor m.

Cut ends tendons of
superficial flaxor m.

Plantar annular ligs.

b.

Abductor digiti
minimi m.

Short digital
flexor tendons

Short digital
flexor m.

Lumbrical
mm.

Digital
anular ligs.

Structures Related to the Claw

PLATE 22

Figure 1.
Medial view of forepaw

Figure 2.
Structures that extend and retract claw. Color the anatomical components responsible for these actions.

1. **Superficial digital flexor tendon**
2. **Deep digital flexor tendon**
3. **Proximal phalanx**
4. **Proximal anular ligament**
5. **Proximal digital anular ligament**
6. **Distal digital anular ligament**
7. **Tendon of deep digital flexor m.**
8. **Middle phalanx**
9. **Distal phalanx**
10. **Claw covering ungual process**
11. **Dorsal elastic ligament**
12. **Combined extensor tendons**
13. **Extensor bands of interossei mm.**
14. **Sesamoid bone**
15. **Common digital extensor tendon**

Figure 1.

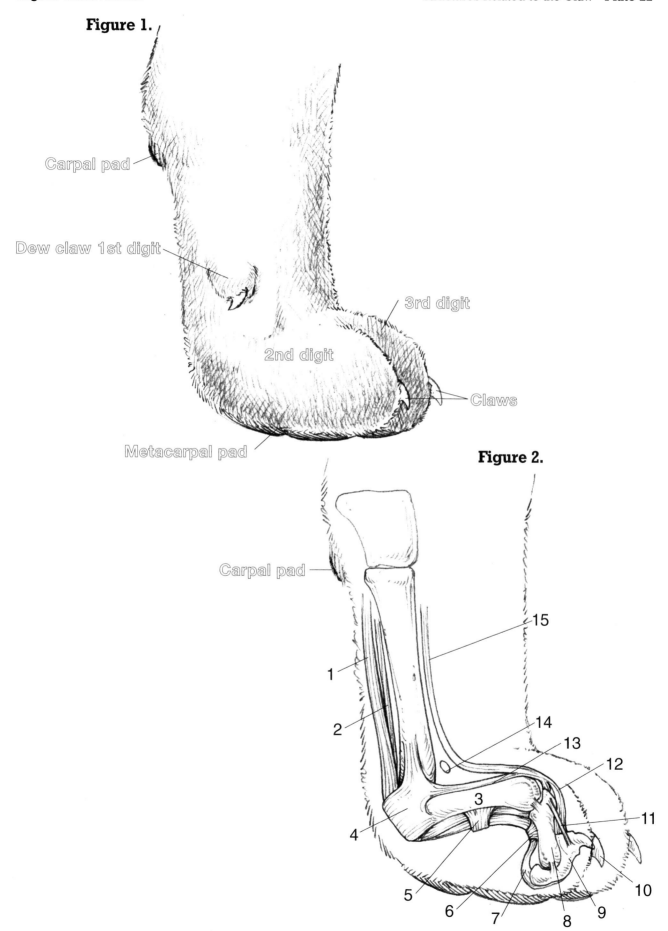

Carpal pad

Dew claw 1st digit

3rd digit

2nd digit

Claws

Metacarpal pad

Figure 2.

Carpal pad

15

1

2

14

13

12

3

11

4

10

5

6   7   8   9

Bones of the Pelvis

PLATE 23

Figure 1. Dorsocaudal view of bony pelvis.

Color in the names of the bones and the bones indicated.

Each **hip bone** (os coxae) consists of the fused **ilium, ischium** (pronounced iskium), **pubis** and **acetabular bone**. The two hip bones are joined at the **pelvic symphysis**. The **sacrum** articulates with each **ilium** at a **sacroiliac joint**.

Underline the following names and color the parts of the bones indicated:

Figure 2. Left lateral view of mature bony pelvis.
1. **Crest of ilium**
2. **Cranial dorsal iliac spine**
3. **Caudal dorsal iliac spine**
4. **Iliopubic eminence**
5. **Ischiatic spine**
6. **Obturator foramen**
7. **Ischiatic tuber**
8. **Pelvic symphysis**
9. **Pecten of pubis**
10. **Sacroiliac joints**
11. **Cranial ventral iliac spine**
12. **Caudal ventral iliac spine**
13. **Acetabulum** - consists of a semicircular articular surface, the lunate face, surrounding a deep acetabular fossa.

Figure 3. Developing **hip bone** of a kitten. Cartilage is stippled. The small **acetabular bone** fuses with the **ilium**, **ischium** and **pubis** to form the **acetabulum** (socket of the hip joint).

Figure 1

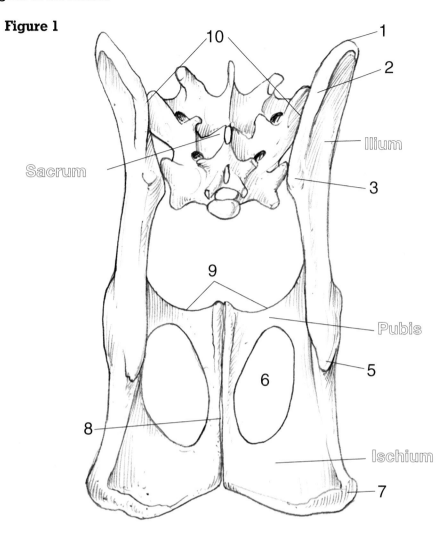

10

1

2

Ilium

Sacrum

3

9

Pubis

5

6

8

Ischium

7

Figure 2

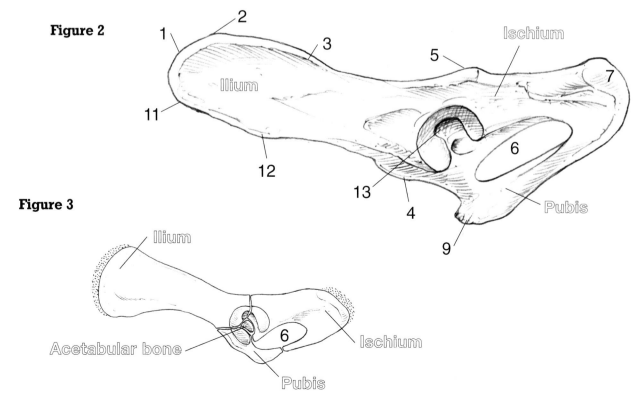

2

1

3

Ischium

5

7

Ilium

11

6

12

13

Pubis

4

9

Figure 3

Ilium

Acetabular bone

6

Ischium

Pubis

Bones of the Thigh and Leg

PLATE 24

Color in the names on the drawing and the bones indicated in different colors.

A. Cranial view of femur. The patella is a large sesamoid bone attached to the femoral quadriceps muscle and its tendon. It slides proximally and distally (up and down) on the trochlea.

B. Caudal view of femur. The ligament of the head of the femur attaches in the fovea. Two small sesamoid bones (fabellae) in the medial and lateral heads of the gastrocnemius muscle articulate with the medial and lateral condyles of the femur. A third even smaller sesamoid bone is in the tendon of origin of the popliteal muscle and articulates with the lateral condyle.

C. Cranial view of tibia and fibula.

D. Caudal view of tibia and fibula.

Underline names and color the following parts of the:

Femur
1. Head
2. Neck
3. Lesser trochanter
4. Greater trochanter
5. Trochlea
6. Medial epicondyle
7. Lateral epicondyle
8. Fovea
9. Trochanteric fossa
10. Intertrochanteric crest
11. Supracondylar tuberosities
12. Lateral condyle
13. Medial condyle

Tibia and **Fibula**
14. Medial condyle
15. Intercondylar eminence
16. Lateral condyle
17. Tibial tuberosity
18. Extensor groove
19. Head of fibula
20. Medial malleolus
21. Lateral malleolus
22. Cochlea

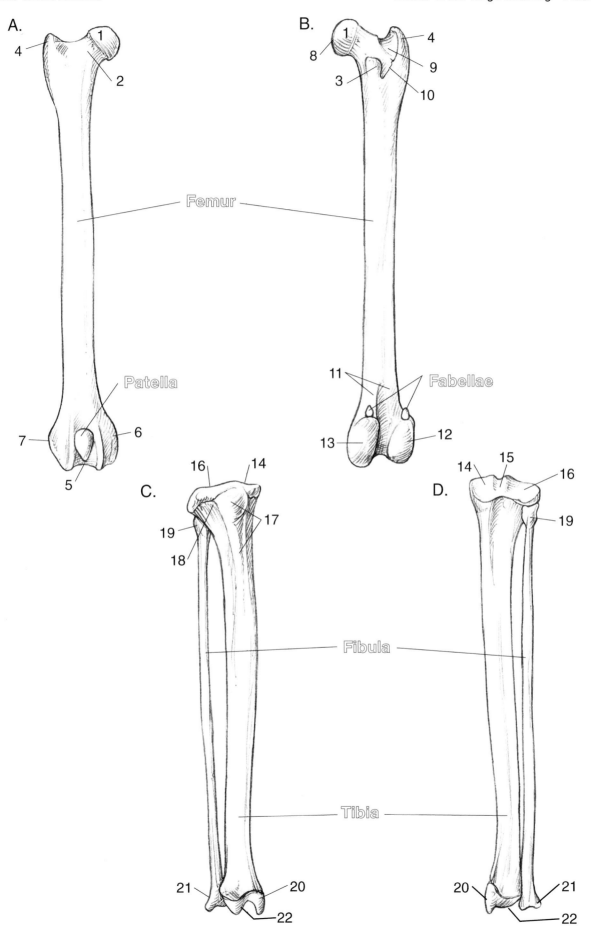

A.

B.

Femur

Patella

Fabellae

C.

D.

Fibula

Tibia

Bones of the Tarsus

PLATE 25

Dorsal, plantar and medial views of the bones of the right tarsus.

There are seven bones in the tarsus (hock): **Fibular tarsal bone** (calcaneus), **tibial tarsal bone** (talus), **central tarsal bone** and the **first, second, third** and **fourth tarsal bones**. More than three times as long as the carpus, the hock includes the talocrural joint between the cochlea of the **tibia** and the **trochlea** of the **tibial tarsal bone** and tarsometatarsal joints between **tarsal bones I** to **IV** and **metatarsal bones I** to **V**.

Except for the shape of the first metatarsal bone and the usual absence of a first digit, the metatarsal bones and phalanges are similar to the metacarpal bones and phalanges of the forefoot (See Plate 26).

Underline the following names and color the bones and their parts:

Calcaneus
Calcaneal tuber
Talus
CT. Central tarsal bone
I. First tarsal bone
II. Second tarsal bone
III. Third tarsal bone
IV. Fourth tarsal bone
I. First metatarsal bone (rudimentary)
II. Second metatarsal bone
III. Third metatarsal bone
IV. Fourth metatarsal bone
V. Fifth metatarsal bone

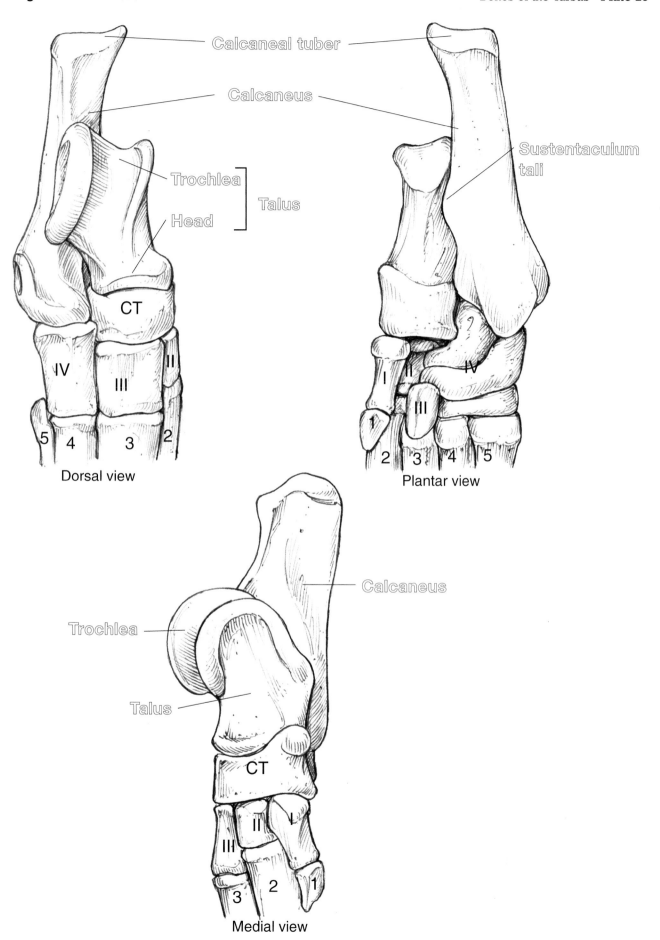

Calcaneal tuber

Calcaneus

Trochlea

Head

Talus

Sustentaculum tali

CT

IV

III

II

5   4   3   2

Dorsal view

I   II

1

III

IV

2   3   4   5

Plantar view

Calcaneus

Trochlea

Talus

CT

II   I

III

3   2   1

Medial view

Tarsal, Metatarsal, and Digital Bones (Phalanges)

PLATE 26

Dorsal view of disarticulated left **tarsal, metatarsal bones** and **phalanges**.

Using different colors, underline the following names and the bones of the tarsus, metatarsus and the digits.

Tal. Talus
Cal. Calcaneus
CT. Central tarsal bone
1. First tarsal bone
2. Second tarsal bone
3. Third tarsal bone
4. Fourth tarsal bone
5. Sesamoid bones
I. First metatarsal bone (rudimentary)
II. Second metatarsal bone
III. Third metatarsal bone
IV. Fourth metatarsal bone
V. Fifth metatarsal bone
1P2, 2P2, 3P2 - First, second and third phalanges of digit 2
1P3, 2P3, 3P3 - First, second and third phalanges of digit 3
1P4, 2P4, 3P4 - First, second and third phalanges of digit 4
1P5, 2P5, 3P5 - First, second and third phalanges of digit 5

Dorsal view

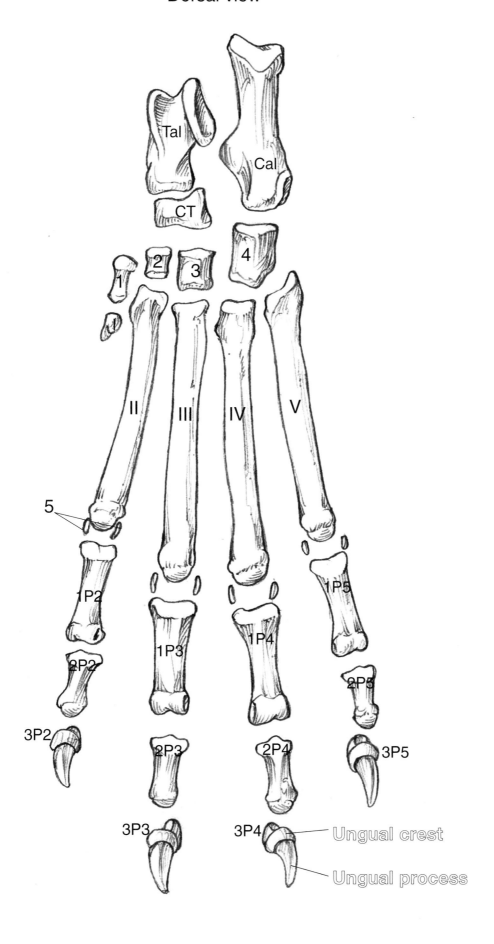

Tal

Cal

CT

2　3　4

1

II　III　IV　V

5

1P2

1P5

1P3　1P4

2P2

2P5

3P2

2P3　2P4　3P5

3P3　3P4

Ungual crest

Ungual process

Joints of the Hindlimb

PLATE 27

Color in the names of the joints. The angles become smaller when the joints are flexed.

The **sacroiliac joint** on each side is formed by articular surfaces on the wing of the ilium and the wing of the sacrum. It is a <u>stabilizing joint</u> in which the articular surfaces are covered with fibrocartilage and supported by <u>dorsal</u> and <u>ventral sacroiliac ligaments</u>.

Among the joints of the hock, the greatest movement occurs in the **tarsocrural joint**. There is some movement between the talus and calcaneus, but very little movement occurs in the **inter-tarsal** and **tarsometatarsal joints**.

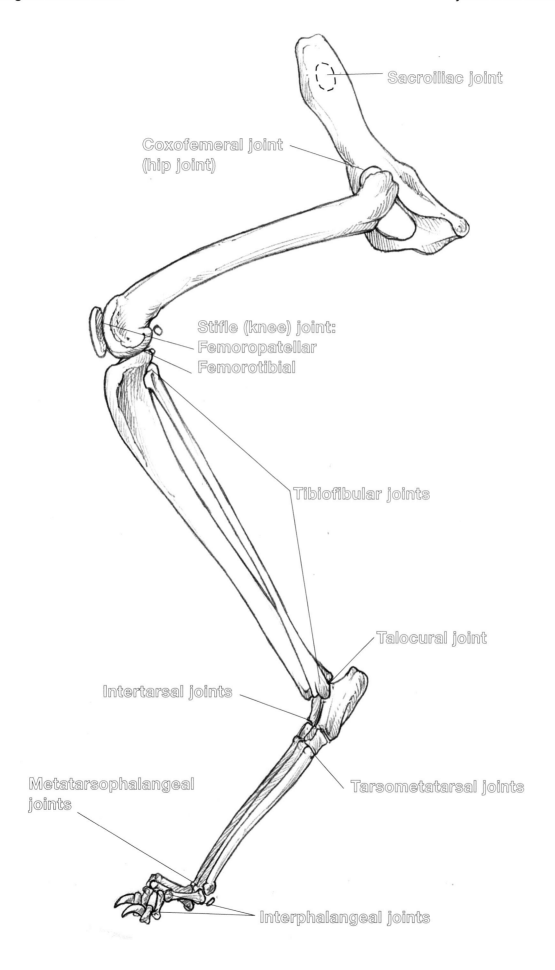

Sacroiliac joint

Coxofemeral joint
(hip joint)

Stifle (knee) joint:
Femoropatellar
Femorotibial

Tibiofibular joints

Talocural joint

Intertarsal joints

Metatarsophalangeal
joints

Tarsometatarsal joints

Interphalangeal joints

Hip Joint

PLATE 28

Ventral view of a cat's bony pelvis and hip joints, including major ligaments.

Using different colors, color the terms and the structures indicated.

Most ligaments function in holding bones together in joints.

These **hip joints** (coxofemoral joints) are normal. The **ligament of the femoral head** binds the head of the femur to the acetabulum. The **transverse acetabular ligament** bridges the notch in the acetabulum, completing the fibrocartilaginous acetabular lip.

Hip dysplasia (from the Greek, dys-, abnormal + plassein, to form) is a relatively common complaint in dogs, but until recently was almost unheard of in the cat. It is a defect of the hip joint, most specifically a failure of the head of the femur (thigh bone) to fit properly into the joint socket, called the acetabulum (pronounced ass-uh-tab-u-lum). If the fit is not tight, the two surfaces rub against each other excessively, causing pain, and eventually osteoarthritis. If the muscles do not have sufficient strength to maintain the fit between the acetabulum and the femoral head, dysplasia will occur.

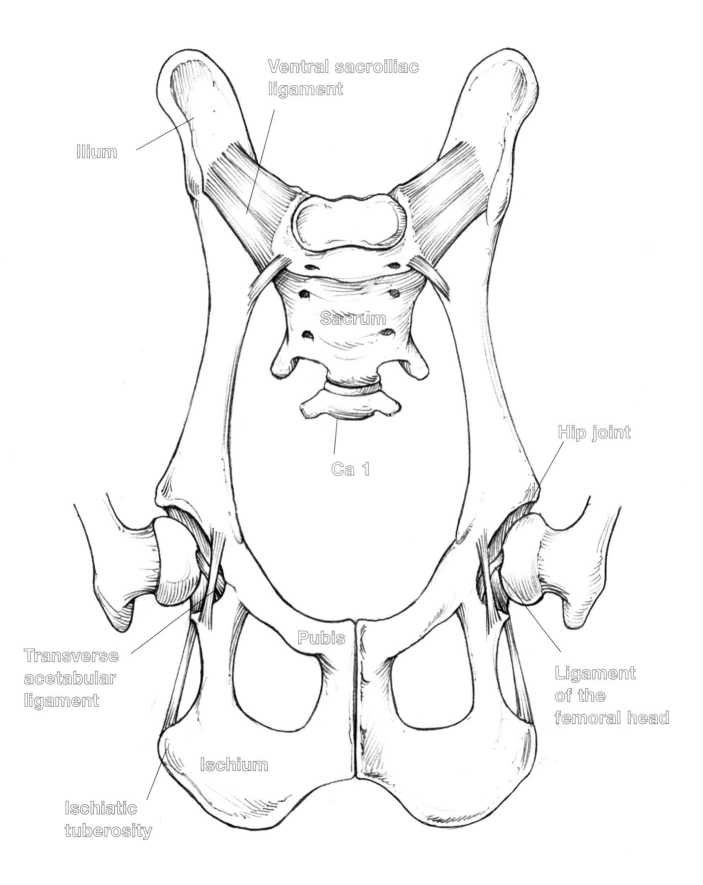

Ventral sacroiliac ligament

Ilium

Sacrum

Ca 1

Hip joint

Transverse acetabular ligament

Pubis

Ligament of the femoral head

Ischium

Ischiatic tuberosity

Stifle Joint

PLATE 29

Dissections of a cat's left stifle joint.
A. Medial view **B.** Lateral view
C. Cranial view **D.** Caudal view

Underline the following terms and color the structures indicated on the drawing.

1. **Tendon - fem. quadriceps m.**
2. **Patella**
3. **Patellar ligament**
   (continues tendon of **fem. quadriceps m.** to **4.**)
4. **Tibial tuberosity**
5. **Sesamoid bones**
6. **Medial meniscus**
7. **Medial collateral ligament**
8. **Tendon - long dig. ext. m.**
9. **Lateral meniscus**
10. **Lateral collateral ligament**
11. **Tendon - popliteal muscle**
12. **Cranial cruciate ligament**
13. **Transverse ligament**
14. **Caudal cruciate ligament**
15. **Meniscofemoral ligament**
16. **Meniscofibular ligament**

There are two joints in the stifle - the femoropatellar joint and the femorotibial joint. A single, compartmented joint capsule is common to both joints. The **patella** is a large sesamoid bone in the **tendon of the femoral quadriceps m.** with the continuing **patellar ligament** attaching to the **tibial tuberosity**. The patella riding on the trochlea of the femur changes direction of pull by the femoral quadriceps muscle, resulting in extension of the femorotibial joint.

Medial and **lateral menisci** (plural of meniscus) are C-shaped plates of fibrocartilage between the femoral condyles and the tibial condyles, providing more congruent articular surfaces.

Named for their tibial attachments, **cranial** and **caudal cruciate ligaments** cross each other as they extend from the femur to the tibia.

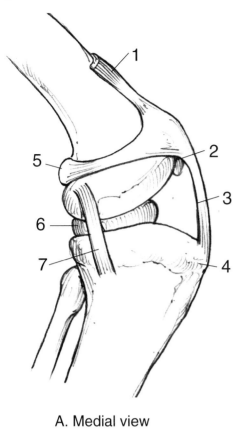

A. Medial view

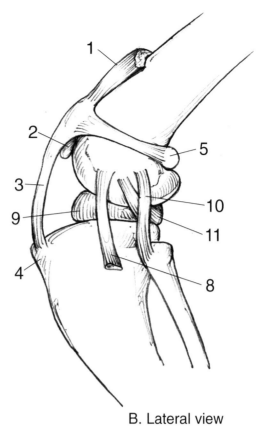

B. Lateral view

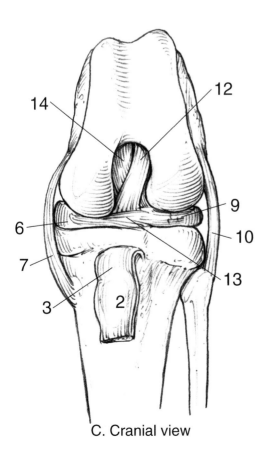

C. Cranial view

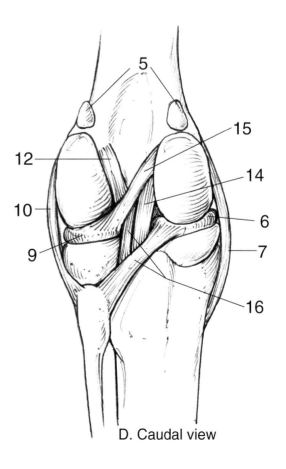

D. Caudal view

Hindlimb Muscles - Lateral Views

PLATE 30

Figure 1. Lateral view of superficial muscles of left hip and thigh.
Figure 2. Lateral view of deep dissection of left hindlimb muscles.

As you color the muscles, try to determine their actions from their positions and the joints they cross. See below.

1. Sartorius m.
2. Tensor fasciae latae m.
3. Middle gluteal m.
4. Superficial gluteal m.
5. Gluteofemoral m.
6. Caudal crural abductor m.
7. sacrocaudalis dorsalis lateralis m.
8. sacrocaudalis ventralis lateralis m.
9. Biceps femoris m.

10. Semitendenosus m.
11. Semimembranosus m.
12. Gastrocnemius m
13. Superficial digital flexor m.
14. Rectus femoris m.
15. Vastus lateralis m.
16. Adductor m.
17. Cranial tibial m.
18. Fibularis longus m.
19. Long digital extensor m.
20. Fibularis brevis m.

The gluteal group of muscles (**superficial, middle** and **deep gluteal muscles** and the **tensor of the fascia lata**) extend the hip and help abduct the hip joint. Insertions of the hamstring group (**femoral biceps, semitendinous** and **semimembranous muscles**) attach proximal and distal to the stifle joint. Tendons from the femoral biceps and semitendinous muscles join tendons of the **superficial digital flexor** and **gastocnemius** to form the **common calcanean tendon**. The main action of the hamstring group is extension of the hip joint. Depending on the location of the muscles and the position of the foot on or off the ground, other actions are flexion or extension of the stifle and extension of the hock. The **internal obturator** and **gemelli muscles** rotate the hip outward. The **long fibular muscle** flexes the hock and turns the foot outward. The **cranial tibial muscle** also flexes the hock but turns the foot inward.

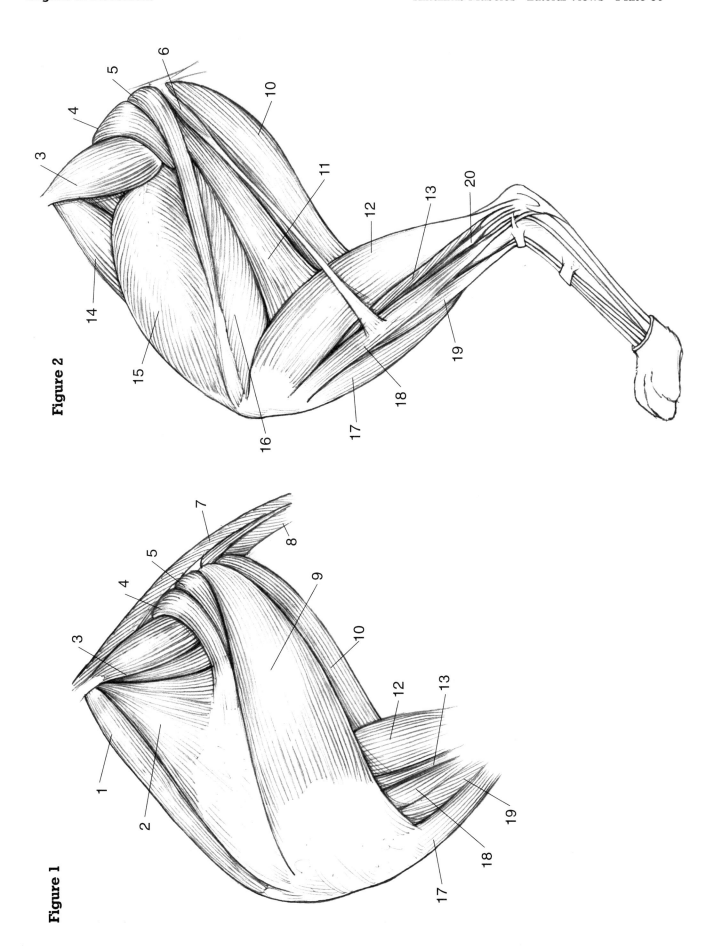

Figure 2

Figure 1

Hindlimb Muscles - Medial Views

PLATE 31

Figure 1. Medial view of superficial muscles of left hindlimb.
Figure 2. Medial view of deep muscles of left hindlimb. m. = muscle.

As you color the muscles indicated, try to visualize their actions from their positions and the joints that they cross. See paragraph below.

1. Femoral triangle
2. Ilioposas m.
3. Pectineus m.
4. Adductor m.
5. Rectus femoris m.
6. Sartorial m.
7. Vastus medialis m.
8. Gracilis m.

9. Semimembranous m.
10. Semitendinous m.
11. Tensor fascia lata m.
12. Gastrocnemius m.
13. Deep digital flexor m.
14. Cranial tibial m.
15. Calcanean tendon

Inserting on the tibial tuberosity by means of the patellar ligament, the four-headed **femoral quadriceps muscle** is the principal extensor of the stifle. The cranial part of the **sartorial muscle** and the cranial part of the **semimembranous muscle** also extend the stifle. Flexors of the stifle include the caudal part of the **sartorial muscle**, the caudal part of the **semimembranous muscle**, and the **semitendinous, gracilis, popliteal** and **gastrocnemius muscles.** Adduction of the hindlimb is done by the **pectineal, adductor** and **gracilis muscles.**

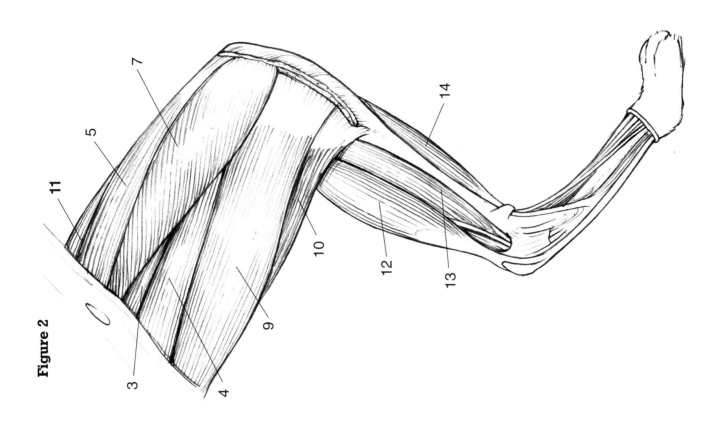

Figure 2

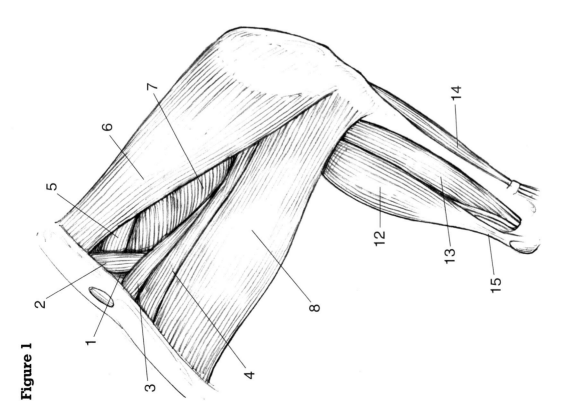

Figure 1

Hindlimb Nerves

PLATE 32

Hindlimb nerves arise from the **lumbosacral plexus** formed by the ventral branches of the last four lumbar nerves and the three sacral nerves. In addition to contributing to hindlimb nerves, sacral nerves also give origin to nerves supplying pelvic organs.

Lateral view of right hindlimb skeleton with courses of nerves related roughly to regions of the hindlimb. Underline the names below and trace the course of each nerve in a different color. n. = nerve

1. **Femoral n.** - To sublumbar muscles and femoral quadriceps m.

2. **Obturator n.** - To adductor muscles of hip

3. **Caudal gluteal n.** - To superficial gluteal m. & part of femoral biceps m.

4. **Cranial gluteal n.** - To middle & deep gluteal & tensor of fascia lata mm.

5. **Pudendal n.** - To urethral sphincter & ischiorectal mm.

6. **Perineal n.** - Sensory to skin of perineum, scrotum & labia and to penis or clitoris

7. **Sciatic n.** - Motor to hamstring muscles Sensory to coxofemoral joint and hindlimb via its branches.

8. **Saphenous n.** -To sartorius m. Sensory to skin of medial thigh

9. **Common fibular n.** - To cranial tibial, digital extensor and peroneal mm. Sensory to stifle joint, skin of lateral crus, dorsal tarsus, metatarsus & digits

10. **Caudal cutaneous sural n.** - Sensory to caudal skin of leg and hock

11. **Superficial fibular n.** - To lat. dig. ext. m.; sensory to skin of leg & foot

12. **Lateral cutaneous sural n.** - sensory to skin of lateral leg.

13. **Deep fibular n.** - to dorsolateral muscles of leg; sensory to foot.

14. **Tibial n.** - to hamstring, gastrocnemius, popliteal and caudal crural mm.

15. **Medial plantar n.** - to medial aspect of foot

16. **Lateral plantar n.** - to lateral and middle aspects of foot

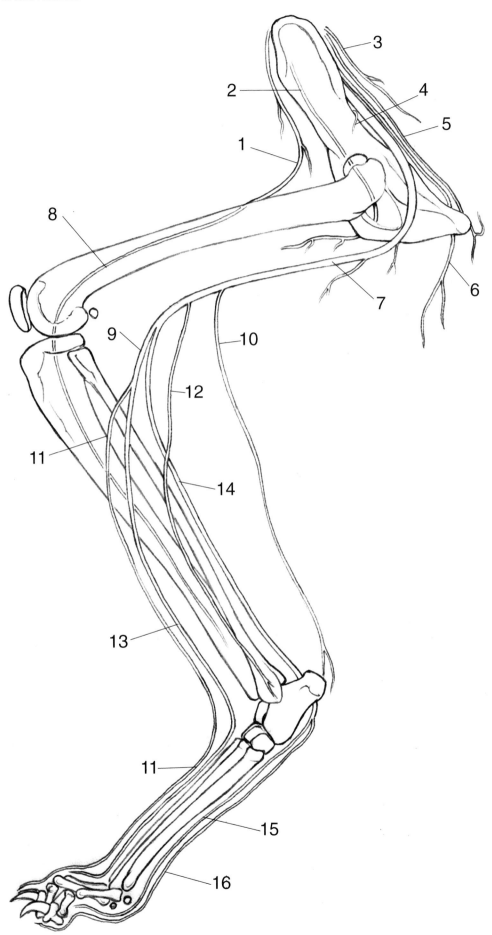

Hindlimb Blood Vessels

PLATE 33

Blood flows to the <u>metatarsal</u> and <u>digital arteries</u> of the hindfoot primarily through the following sequence of arteries: **external iliac - femoral - popliteal - cranial tibial - dorsal pedal**.

Branches of the **saphenous a.** supply the skin: the caudal branch gives origin to the **lateral plantar a.** and **plantar common digital aa.** The anterior branch gives rise to the **medial plantar a.** and **dorsal common digital aa.**

Most veins are satellites (Latin, *satelles* = an attendant) of arteries.

1. **Cranial gluteal a.**
2. **Caudal gluteal a.**
3. **Caudal epigastric a.**
4. **lateralcircumflex femoral a.**
5. **External pudental a.**
6. **Internal pudental a.**

7. **Medial circumflex femoral a.**
8. **Descending genicular a.**
9. **Distal caudal femoral a.**
10. **Saphenous a.**
11. **Cranial br. saphenous a.**
12. **Caudal br. saphenous a.**
13. **Superficial br. crainial tibial a.**

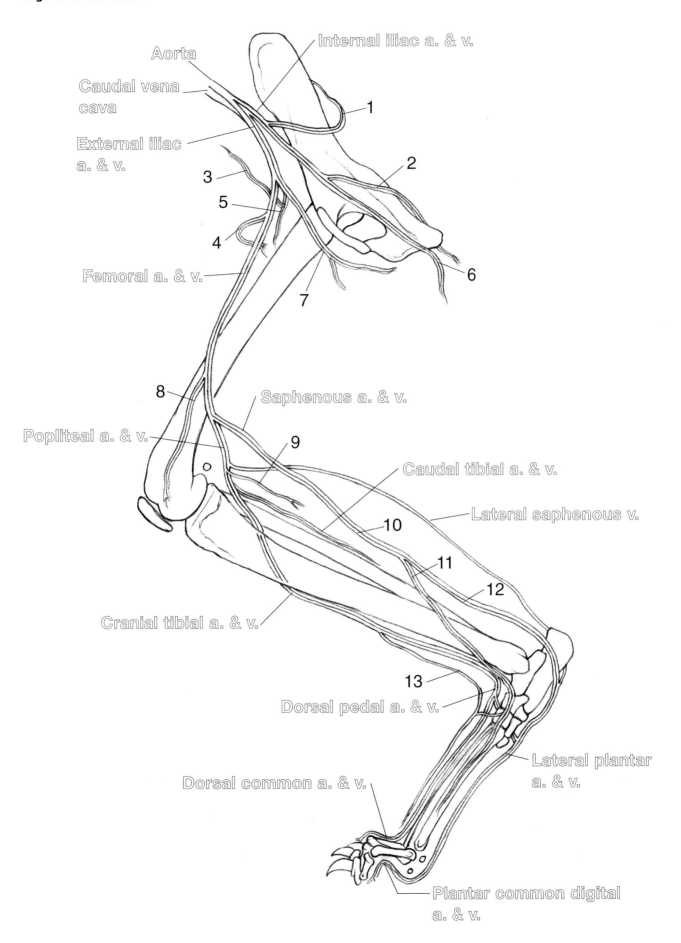

Internal iliac a. & v.

Aorta

Caudal vena cava

External iliac a. & v.

Femoral a. & v.

Saphenous a. & v.

Popliteal a. & v.

Caudal tibial a. & v.

Lateral saphenous v.

Cranial tibial a. & v.

Dorsal pedal a. & v.

Lateral plantar a. & v.

Dorsal common a. & v.

Plantar common digital a. & v.

1

2

3

4

5

6

7

8

9

10

11

12

13

Back and Neck Muscles

PLATE 34

Figure 1. Epaxial muscle systems. Lateral views.

Using three different colors, fill in the diagrammatic drawings of the:

   I. Iliocostal muscle system - lateral group of muscles
      1. Thoracic iliocostal m.
      2. Lumbar Iliocostal m.

  II. Longest (Longissimus) muscle system - intermediate group of muscles
      3. Longest capital (head) m.
      4. Longest cervical m.
      5. Longest thoracic and lumbar m.

 III. Transversospinal muscle system - medial group of muscles
      6. Capital semispinal m. - formed by the two muscles below.
        a. Cervical biventer m.
        b. Complex m.
      7. Splenius m. (cut and reflected)
      8. Spinal and semispinal muscles

      Multifidus and rotator muscles – not seen here; deeper, between vertebrae

Epaxial muscles lie dorsal to the vertebral transverse processes. Working together, they extend the neck and back; on one side, they produce lateral movement. Hypaxial muscles are located ventral to the vertebral bodies and tranverse processes.

Figure 2. Sublumbar muscles (ventral to last three thoracic and the lumbar vertebrae).
Ventral view of muscles on the right side. Also considered with muscles of the pelvic limb.
    1. Lumbar quadrate m. – fixes lumbar vertebral column
    2. Minor psoas m. – flexes lumbar vertebral column
    3. Major psoas m.
    4. Iliacus m. - This muscle and the **major psoas m.** fuse to form the **iliopsoas m.**, the primary flexor of the hip. If the femur is fixed, it flexes the vertebral column. If the pelvic limb is extended caudad, the trunk is pulled caudad.

Figure 1

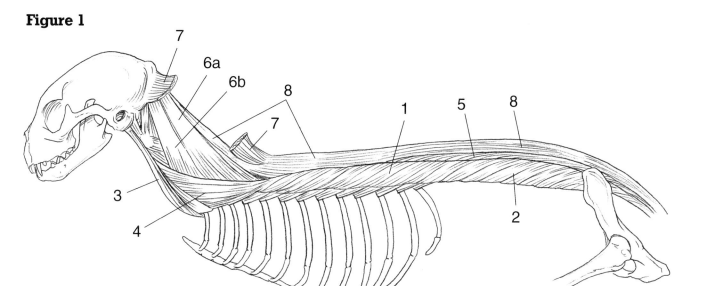

Figure 2

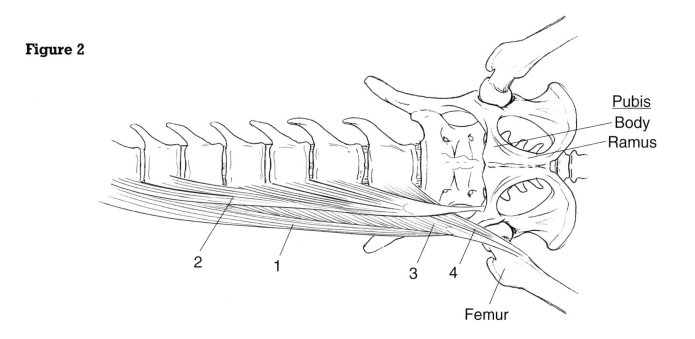

Tails

PLATE 35

Figure 1. Tail muscles.

Locate and color the tail muscles. m. = muscle.

The cat's tail is elevated (extended) by contraction of the **medial** and **lateral dorsal sacrocaudal muscles**; the tail is depressed (flexed) by the **medial** and **lateral ventral sacrocaudal muscles**; and it is flexed laterad (to the side by the **caudal intertransverse**, **anal levator** and **coccygeal muscles**.

Figure 2. Types of tails. Color the tails and their names.

Type of Tail	Examples
Bushy	**Maine Coon**
Bobtail	**Japanese Bobtail**
Regular	**Russian Blue**
No tail	**Manx**

Figure 1

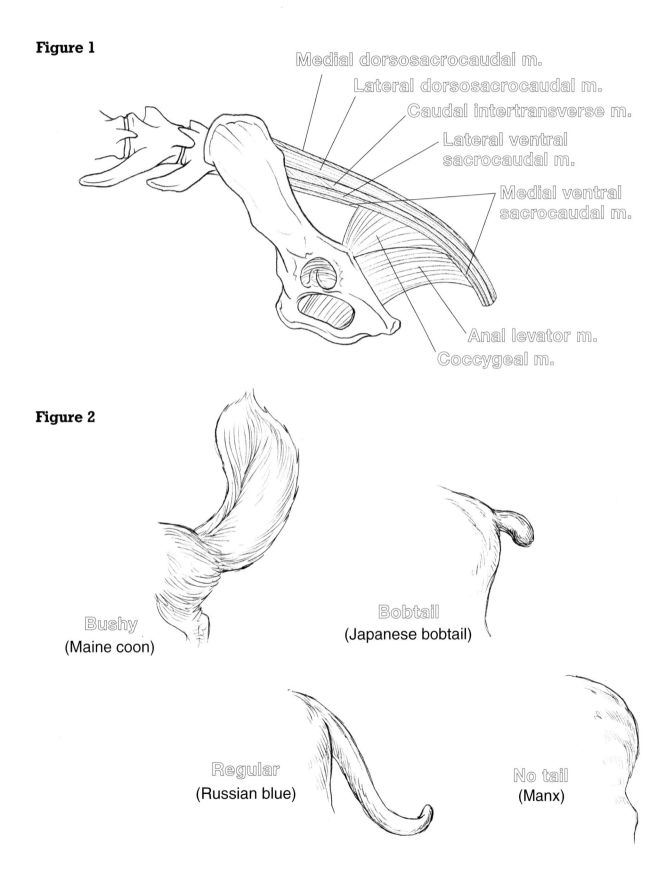

Medial dorsosacrocaudal m.

Lateral dorsosacrocaudal m.

Caudal intertransverse m.

Lateral ventral sacrocaudal m.

Medial ventral sacrocaudal m.

Anal levator m.

Coccygeal m.

Figure 2

Bushy
(Maine coon)

Bobtail
(Japanese bobtail)

Regular
(Russian blue)

No tail
(Manx)

Body Types

PLATE 36

Breeding cats started in the 19th century mainly in Britain. There are about 100 recognized pedigree breeds today; those cats that are non-pedigree are termed moggie. Pedigree and moggie cats have a great verity of hair coats and color patterns, but they generally fall into three main body types:

Figure 1. Cobby type: compact, heavy-set body, short legs, broad head, and large round eyes.

Figure 2. Muscular type: sturdy-muscular body with round full – cheeked head.

Figure 3. Foreign type: slender body, long legs and tail, triangular shaped head, long ears, and slanting eyes.

Color typical patterns or solid color on body types.

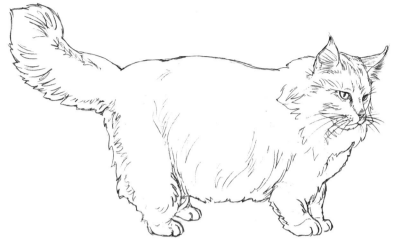
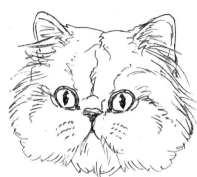

Figure 1. Cobby type (Persian)

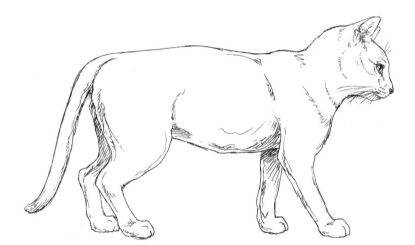
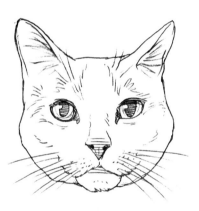

Figure 2. Muscular type (American shorthair)

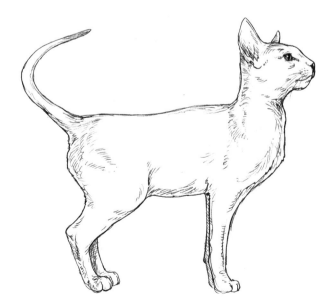
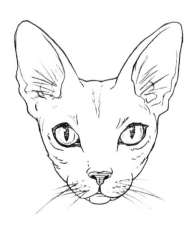

Figure 3. Foreign type (Sphynx)

The Head

The Skull and Associated Bones

PLATE 37

Figure 1. Lateral view of skull, mandible and hyoid apparatus.

Figure 2. Dorsal view of skull.

Color in the labels and the bones that they indicate.
Underline the following parts of bones and identify them on the drawings:

1. **External occipital protuberance**
2. **Nuchal crest**
3. **Occipital condyle**
4. **Jugular process**
5. **Tympanic bulla**
6. **External acoustic meatus**
7. **Zygomatic arch**
8. **Coronoid process**
   (of mandible)

9. **Temporomandibular joint**
10. **Angular process**
11. **Mandibular foramen**
    (on medial side)
12. **Mental foramina**
13. **Infraorbital foramen**
14. **Sagittal crest**
15. **Zygomatic process**

Since sutures are fibrous joints that ossify with age, junctions between most bones of the skull become indistinct. They are all ossified by 4 years of age.

The inner end of the **external acoustic meatus** is covered by the eardrum (tympanic membrane). The **tympanic bulla** covers the middle ear, and the inner ear is contained within the petrous part of the **temporal bone**.

The **hyoid apparatus** consists of nine small bones and two cartilages that attach to the skull. This arrangement of bones joins the skull to the thyroid cartilage of the larynx and the base of the tongue in which the unpaired basihyoid bone is embedded.

Figure 1

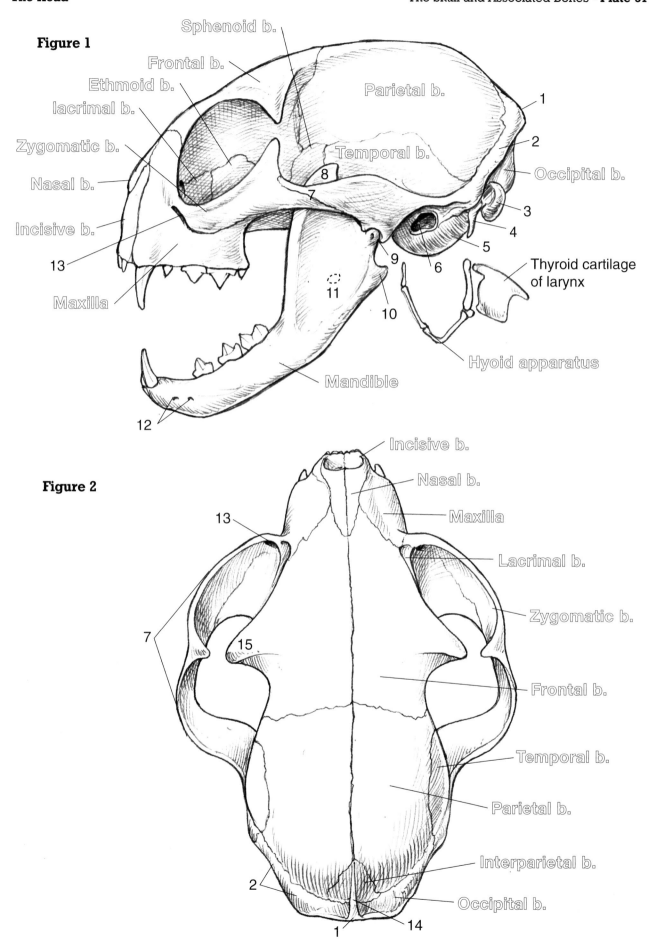

Sphenoid b.

Frontal b.

Ethmoid b.

lacrimal b.

Zygomatic b.

Nasal b.

Incisive b.

Parietal b.

Temporal b.

1

2

Occipital b.

3

4

5

6

8

7

9

13

Maxilla

11

10

Thyroid cartilage of larynx

12

Hyoid apparatus

Mandible

Figure 2

Incisive b.

Nasal b.

Maxilla

13

Lacrimal b.

Zygomatic b.

7

15

Frontal b.

Temporal b.

Parietal b.

Interparietal b.

2

Occipital b.

1

14

Cavities and Openings in the Skull

PLATE 38

Figure 1. Ventral view of skull.
Figure 2. Sagittal (parallel to median plane) view of skull to the right of the nasal septum.
Figure 3. Outline of paranasal sinuses from the exterior.

Color the names and the bones and cavities they label. Underline the following structures and openings and identify them by the numbers on the drawings:

1. Foramen magnum
2. Jugular foramen
3. Jugular process
4. Tympanic bulla
5. Mastoid process
6. External acoustic meatus
7. Round foramen
8. Oval foramen

9. Palatine fissure
10. Bony tentorium of cerebellum
11. External occipital protuberance
12. Hypophyseal fossa
13. Retroarticular process
14. Cribriform plate
15. Dorsal nasal concha
16. Ventral nasal concha

Blood vessels and cranial nerves pass through the foramina (plural of foramen), canals and fissures in the skull. The spinal cord and blood vessels leave the **cranial cavity** through the **foramen magnum**.

A **choana** is the caudal opening of a **nasal fossa**. Left and right halves (nasal fossae) of the **nasal cavity** are separated by the **nasal septum**, a bony, cartilaginous and membranous partition.

Paranasal sinuses are mucous membrane-lined cavities that open into the **nasal cavity** on each side. The **maxillary recess** is not a true sinus because it is not fully enclosed by the maxilla.

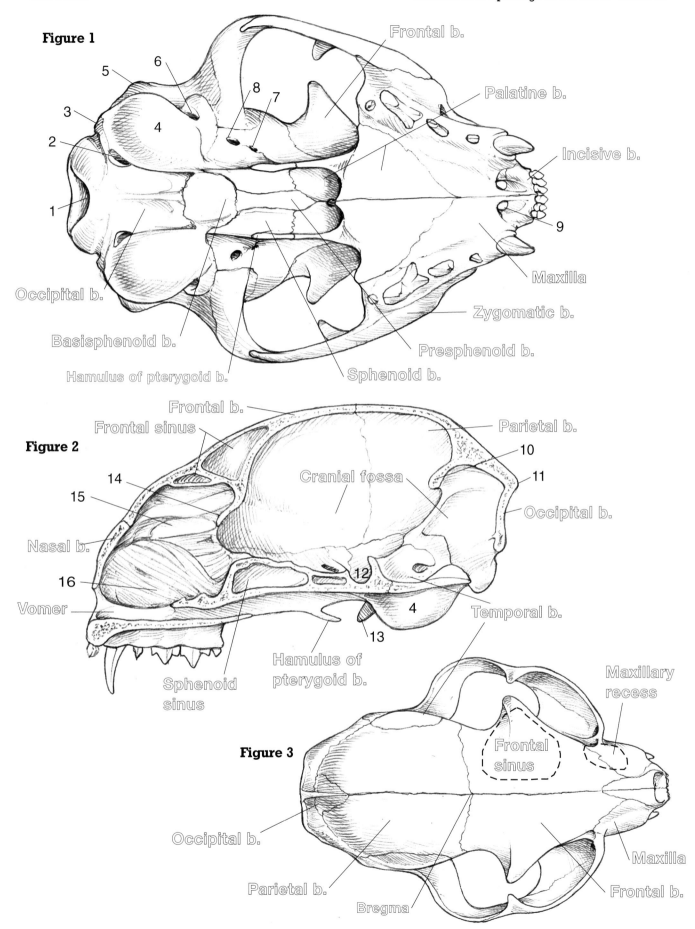

Figure 1

Frontal b.

Palatine b.

Incisive b.

5
6
8
7
3
4
2
1
9

Occipital b.

Maxilla

Basisphenoid b.

Zygomatic b.

Hamulus of pterygoid b.

Presphenoid b.

Sphenoid b.

Figure 2

Frontal b.

Frontal sinus

Parietal b.

10
11

Occipital b.

Cranial fossa

14
15

Nasal b.

16

Vomer

12
13
4

Hamulus of pterygoid b.

Temporal b.

Sphenoid sinus

Figure 3

Maxillary recess

Frontal sinus

Occipital b.

Maxilla

Parietal b.

Bregma

Frontal b.

Lateral Structures of the Head

PLATE 39

Figure 1. Major superficial muscles. Platysma and superficial cervical sphincter muscles removed.
Figure 2. Superficial veins and nerves. Salivary glands.

Underline each boldfaced name in color. Then locate and color the structure labeled on the drawings in the same color. Use blue for veins; yellow for nerves. m. = muscle; v . = vein; n. = nerve.

1. **Mental m.**
2. **Oral orbicular m.** (cut)
3. **Canine m.**
4. **Maxillary lip levator m.**
5. **Nasolabial levator m.** (cut)
6. **Ocular orbicular m.**
7. **Zygomatic major & minor mm.**
8. **Frontal m.**
9. **Zygomaticoauricular m.**
10. **Cervicoauricular muscles**
11. **Temporal m.**
12. **Parotid salivary gland**
13. **Mandibular salivary gland**
14. **External jugular v.**
15. **Parotidoauricular m.**

16. **Mandibular lymph nodes**
17. **Masseter m.**
18. **Deep sphincter m. of neck**
19. **Buccinator m.**
20. **Ocular angular v.**
21. **Dorsal branch of facial n.**
22. **Facial v.**
23. **Parotid duct**
24. **Ventral branch of facial n.**
25. **Second cervical n.**
26. **Great auricular n.**
27. **Maxillary v.**
28. **Linguofacial v.**
29. **Buccal salivary gland**
30. **Buccal lymph node**

Figure 1

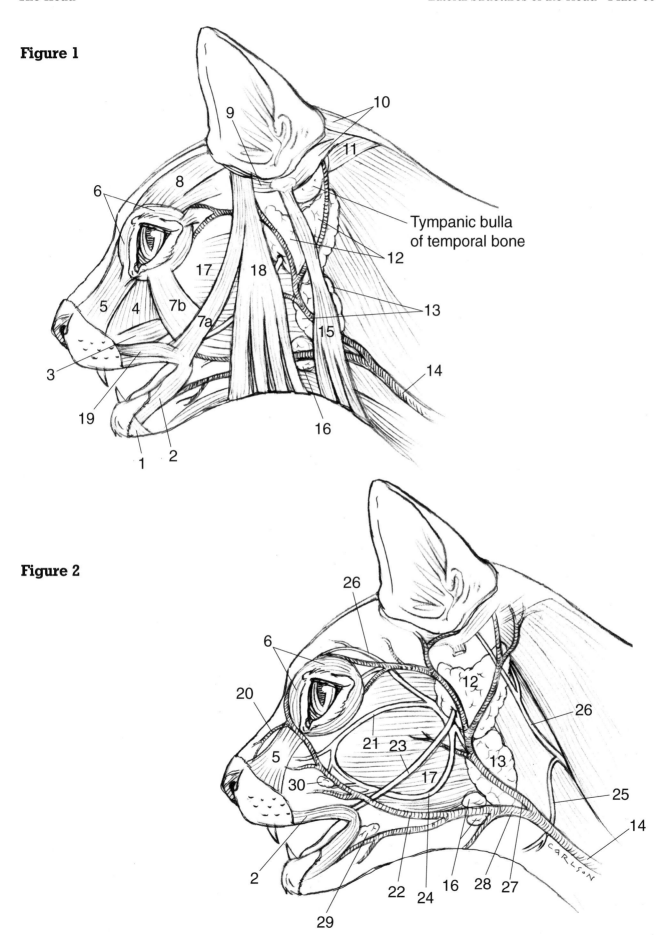

Tympanic bulla
of temporal bone

Figure 2

Ventral Structures of the Head

PLATE 40

Figure 1. Ventral superficial muscles of the head. m. = muscle.
Figure 2. Deeper dissection of ventral aspect of the head.

Underline each **boldfaced name** in a different color. Then locate and color the organ labeled on the drawings in the same color.

1. **Sternocephalic m.**
2. **Sternohyoid m.**
3. **Medial retropharyngeal lymph node**
4. **Basihyoid bone**
5. **Stylohyoid m.**
6. **Digastric m.**
7. **Masseter m.**
8. **Mylohyoid m.**
9. **Sternothyroid m.**
10. **First cervical nerve**
11. **Cranial laryngeal nerve**
12. **Hypoglossal nerve**
13. **Lingual artery**
14. **Hyoglossal m.**
15. **Styloglossal m.**
16. **Geniohyoid m.**
17. **Genioglossal m.**
18. **Common carotid artery**
19. **Vagosympathetic trunk**
20. **Mandibular salivary gland**
21. **Sublingual salivary gland**
22. **Major sublingual duct**
23. **Mandibular duct**

Of special significance in Figure 2 are the **hypoglossal nerve**, the motor supply to the muscles of the tongue, the **lingual artery**, and the **mandibular** and **sublingual glands** and their ducts. The **vagosympathetic nerve trunk** (alongside the **common carotid artery**) carries autonomic nerve fibers from and to the head.

Figure 1

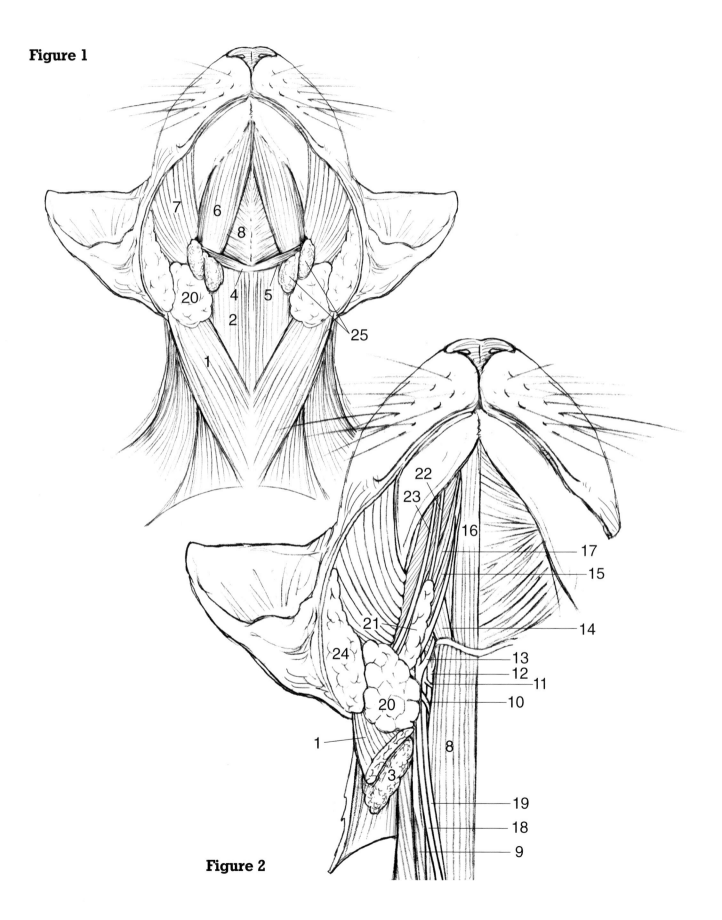

Figure 2

The Eye and Accessory Ocular Structures

PLATE 41

Figure 1. The visible eye and accessory structures. Deeper structures outlined.
Figure 2. Course of the flow of tears. Trace the structures involved.
Figure 3. Sagittal section of the eye.

Underline each **boldfaced term** below in a different color. Then color the structure labeled on the drawing in the same color.

1. Reflection of **conjunctiva** - lining of eyelids and anterior eye. Color dotted line.
2. **Lacrimal gland** - secretes tears.
3. **Lateral commissure** - junction of palpebrae (L., eyelids).
4. **Sclera** - fibrous "white of eye".
5. **Iris** - Looking through cornea, C. Muscles control size of pupil.
6. **Pupil** – opening in 5.
7. **Tarsal gland openings** - dots. Lower palpebra pulled down.
8. **Third eyelid** - cartilage outlined.
9. **Gland of 3rd eyelid** -secretes part of the tear film.
10. **Lacrimal caruncle** - an elevation
11. **Lacrimal punctum** - opening in palpebra, draining tears into **12**.
12. **Lacrimal canaliculi**
13. **Lacrimal sac**
14. **Nasolacrimal duct**
15. **Nasal punctum** of **14**.
16. **Choroid** - vascular layer.
17. **Tapetum** - reflective region in the choroid.
18. **External muscles of eye**
19. **Optic nerve**
20. **Blood vessels to retina**

Color the path of light (arrow) through the transparent parts of the eye: **cornea (C), anterior chamber (A), posterior chamber (P), lens (L), vitreous chamber (V), and retina (R).** Watery aqueous humor fills the anterior and posterior chambers; the jelly-like vitreous body fills the vitreous chamber. The cornea and lens both bend light rays, focusing them on the retina. Light hitting photoreceptive cells in the retina starts a series of nerve impulses in other cells carried to the brain by nerve fibers in the optic nerve.

Cat vision is designed for detecting motion, useful for hunting. Like humans, cats have binocular vision, although not as well tuned as in humans. This means a cat most likely sees in 3-D, as do humans, which is very useful for judging distance.

Cats appear to be slightly nearsighted, which would suggest their vision is tailored more for closer objects, such as prey, that they can capture within running distance.

Cats have an elliptical pupil. It opens and closes much faster than round types and allows for a much larger pupil size. This allows more light to enter the eye. Cats also have a mirror-like membrane in the choroid layer behind the retina called the **tapetum**. It reflects the light passing through the rod cells back through the retina a second time to further stimulate the photoreceptor cells. The result is a double exposure of the light, which permit cats to see well in near darkness. They can see in one-sixth the amount of light that people need.

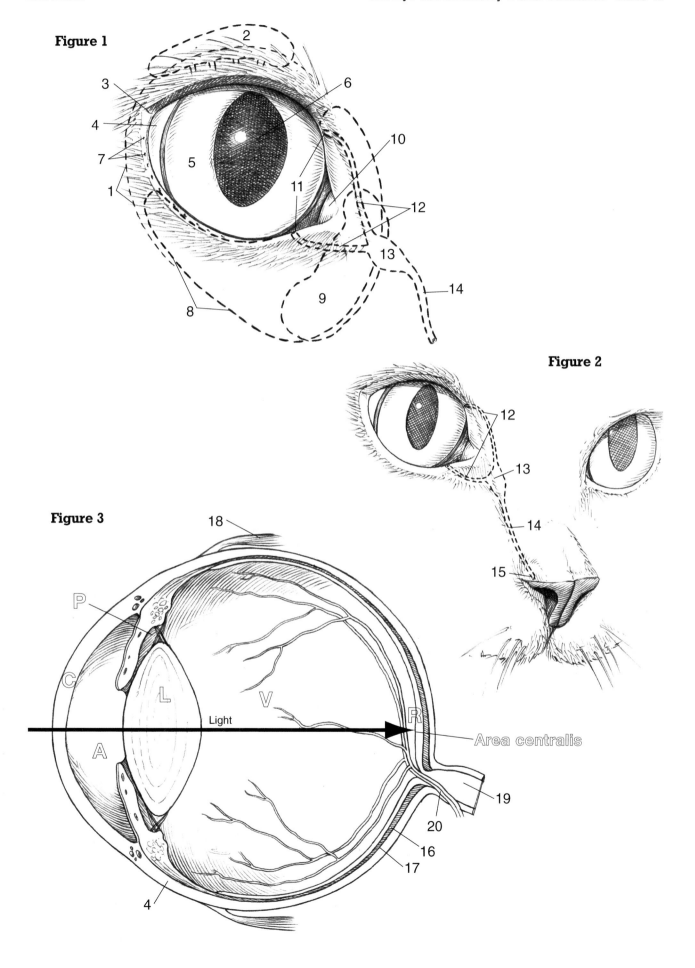

Figure 1

Figure 2

Figure 3

Light

Area centralis

The Nose

PLATE 42

Figure 1. Normal external nose.
Figure 2. Nasal cartilages.
Figure 3. Distribution of olfactory nerves in the mucous membrane of the nasal septum and ethmoturbinates. Sagittal view. Part of the bony nasal septum removed to expose the left ethmoturbinates.

Underline the names below and color the names on the plate different colors.

1. Ethmoturbinates	**7. Nasal cartilages**
2. Cribriform plate of ethmoid b.	**8. Nasal bone**
3. Right olfactory bulb of brain	**9. Incisive duct**
4. Olfactory nerve fibers	**10. Vomeronasal organ**
5. Ethmoidal nerve	**11. Vomeronasal nerves**
6. Nasal septum	**12. Palatine process of maxilla**

Cartilages and attached muscles change the shape of the nostrils. There are no hairs or glands in the normally pigmented skin. The "healthy" cool nose is kept moist by lacrimal and lateral nasal gland secretions. The pattern of ridges in the thick skin here is unique to individual cats. Thus, nose prints are similar to human fingerprints.

Color the names indicated in **bold face**:

An olfactory mucous membrane covers half of **ethmoturbinates** of the ethmoidal labyrinth, the caudal half of the nasal septum, and much of the walls of the caudal nasal cavity. Substances in the nasal secretions stimulate olfactory cells. Their **nerve fibers** pass through the **cribriform plate** to the **olfactory bulbs** of the brain. The **ethmoidal nerve** senses irritation and starts sneezing. A cat's sense of smell (olfaction) is several hundred times more sensitive than that of a human.

Odors of pheromones produced by related individuals or during heat (estrus) in females are detected by olfactory neurons in each **vomeronasal organ** (organ of Jacobsen). Supported by a scroll of cartilage, this tubule of olfactory mucous membrane opens into an **incisive duct** which opens into the nasal cavity and next to the incisive papilla in the oral cavity. In the flehmen response in a male cat, the tongue licks rapidly against the hard palate, the upper lips curl and the mouth opens slightly. This forces pheromone-bearing nasal secretions into the incisive ducts and vomeronasal organs.

Figure 1   A.   B.

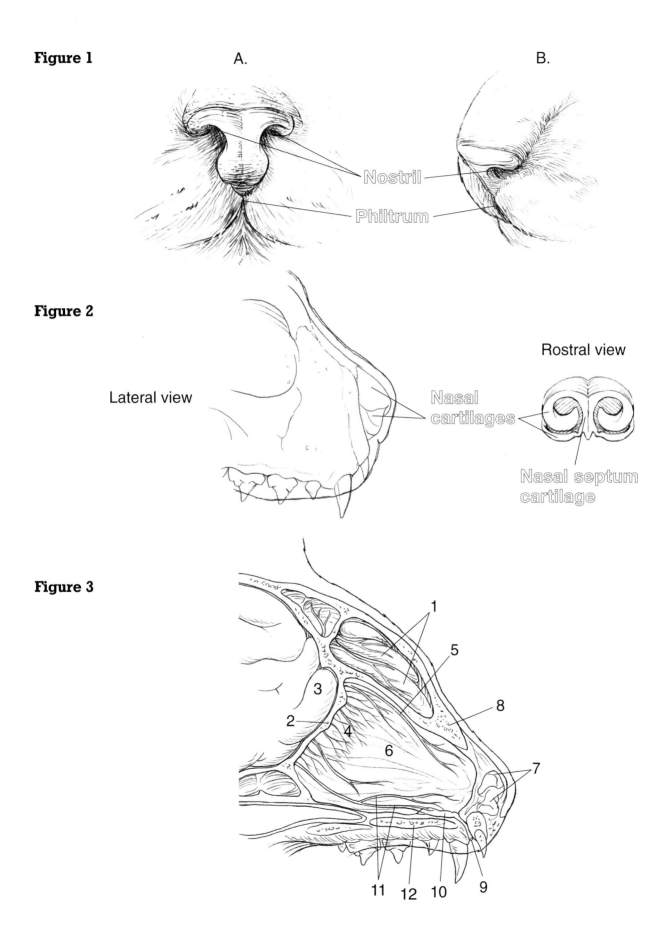

Nostril

Philtrum

Figure 2

Lateral view

Rostral view

Nasal
cartilages

Nasal septum
cartilage

Figure 3

1

5

3

8

2

4

6

7

11   12   10

9

The Ear

PLATE 43

Figure 1. External ear. Drawing of a dissection exposing the ear canal.
Figure 2. Middle ear and inner ear. Schematic drawing of the temporal bone showing the auditory ossicles (little ear bones).

Color the names on the drawings and color the structures where appropriate.

1. **Tympanic membrane**
2. **Malleus (hammer)**
3. **Incus (anvil)**
4. **Stapes (stirrup)**

5. **Vestibule**
6. **Semicircular ducts**
7. **Cochlea**

The cat's **pinna** (containing elastic auricular cartilage) is usually short pointed or long pointed (breeds from warm climates) but may assume a curled or folded shape in some breeds (American Curl, Scottish Fold). Auricular (ear) muscles act independently on each side of the head, directing the pinna toward the sound. Notice the bend between the **vertical ear canal** and the **horizontal ear canal**. Skin lining the ear canal contains many apocrine tubular (sweat) and sebaceous (oil) glands. Their combined secretions forms the dry, brownish cerumen (ear wax). When the ear canal is inflamed by ear mites or an infection, the secretion increases and is more liquid.

An **auditory tube** extends from the nasopharynx to the middle ear, serving to equalize pressure on each side of the eardrum.

Sound waves in the ear canal vibrate the **eardrum**. The **malleus** (partly embedded in the eardrum) **incus** and **stapes** gear down the vibrations and transmit them to a liquid in the inner ear. These vibrations move membranes in the **cochlea** that stimulate hair cells, producing nerve impulses carried to the brain by the vestibulocochlear nerve.

Cats sense of hearing is one of the highest in animal kingdom. Hearing power of cats is about three times greater than human beings; hearing power of cats is about two times greater than dogs. Cats can hear sounds of up to 65kHz; dogs can hear sounds of up to 30kHz; the upper human limit is around 20kHz.

Three bony **semicircular canals** situated at approximately 90 degrees to one another surround membranous **semicircular ducts** containing a liquid that stimulates a sensory region in each canal. These regions are stimulated by changes in the position of the head. Sensory regions in the membranous **utricle** and **saccule** in the bony **vestibule** are stimulated by positive or negative linear acceleration. Nerve impulses from these sensory regions in the membranous labyrinth of the inner ear are carried to the brain by the vestibulocochlear nerve.

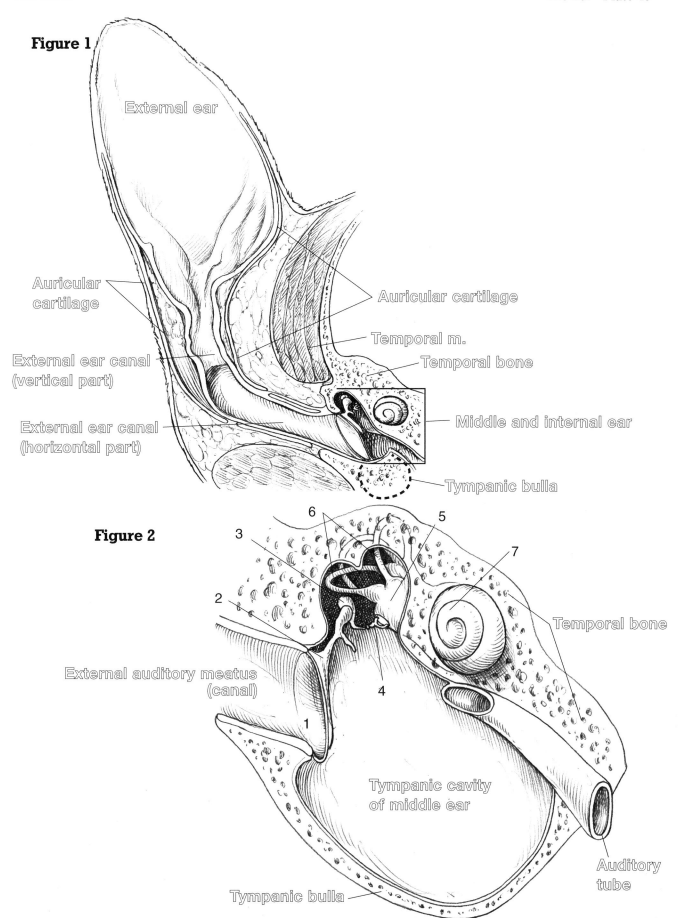

Figure 1

External ear

Auricular
cartilage

Auricular cartilage

Temporal m.

Temporal bone

External ear canal
(vertical part)

External ear canal
(horizontal part)

Middle and internal ear

Tympanic bulla

Figure 2

6

5

3

7

2

Temporal bone

External auditory meatus
(canal)

4

1

Tympanic cavity
of middle ear

Tympanic bulla

Auditory
tube

Digestive System

The Teeth

PLATE 44

Figure 1. The permanent teeth.

Underline the names and abbreviations of the teeth listed below in different colors, and color the teeth as they are labeled on the drawing.

I1 **First incisor tooth**

I2 **Second incisor tooth**

I3 **Third incisor tooth**

C **Canine tooth**

P2 **Second premolar tooth**

P3 **Third premolar tooth**

M1 **First molar tooth**

The dental formula for the cat's permanent teeth: **2(I3/3 C1/1 P3/2 M1/1) = 30**

The teeth of the upper dental arch are lateral to those in the lower dental arch. The lower canine tooth bites rostral to the upper canine. The incisor and canine teeth are used for grasping; the premolars and molars used for cutting.

The usual dental formula for the deciduous teeth: **2(Di3/3 Dc1/1 Dp3/2) = 26**

Figure 2. Longitudinal section through a simple tooth.

On the drawing, underline the names and the structures labeled in different colors.

Periodontal (around the tooth) disease is a common disease of cats. Tooth fracture is the second most common dental problem. Soft llght-colored plaque on the tooth and **gingiva** is composed of food particles, bacteria and deposits of saliva. Minerals in saliva will harden plaque into **tartar (calculus)** that will expand in the **gingival groove**, irritating the gum and causing gingivitis (inflammation of the gums). This leads to periodontitis. Bacteria multiply, causing bleeding and tissue loss, destruction of the periodontal ligament and loosening of the tooth. Inflammation spreads to alveolar bone, causing bone loss and, eventually, loss of the tooth.

Figure 1

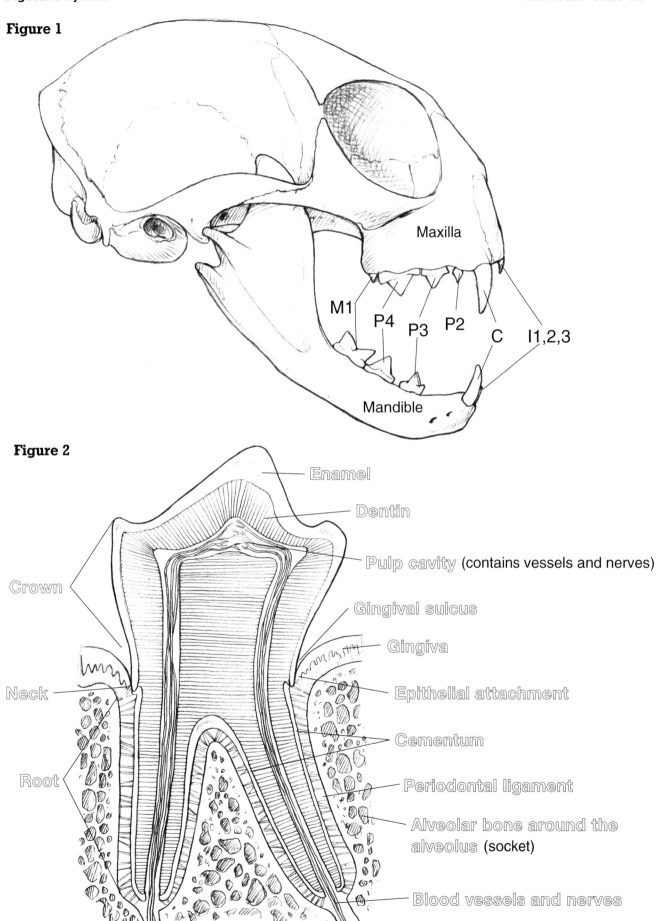

Maxilla

M1

P4

P3

P2

C

I1,2,3

Mandible

Figure 2

Enamel

Dentin

Pulp cavity (contains vessels and nerves)

Gingival sulcus

Gingiva

Crown

Epithelial attachment

Neck

Cementum

Periodontal ligament

Root

Alveolar bone around the alveolus (socket)

Blood vessels and nerves

Salivary Glands

PLATE 45

Dissection of a cat's head exposing the main salivary glands and their ducts. The mandible has been removed.

Color the names on the drawing in different colors and color the labeled organs the same colors.

The **parotid duct** (cut near its origin in this drawing) crosses the masseter muscle and opens into the vestibule (space between the lips and cheeks and the teeth and gums) opposite the upper fourth premolar tooth. The **zygomatic gland** lies just under the orbit. One large and three or four small **zygomatic gland ducts** open into the vestibule caudal to the upper first molar. The **mandibular duct** crosses the **digastric muscle** and then runs along with the **major sublingual duct** from the **monostomatic** (having one opening) **part of the sublingual gland**. The two ducts pass between the genioglossal and mylohyoid muscles and are then enclosed by a sublingual fold of mucous membrane as they extend to their openings on the **sublingual papilla**. Several tiny ducts from the **polystomatic** (having several openings) **part of the sublingual gland** empty into the ventrocaudal vestibule. The salivary glands' secretion, saliva, moistens and lubricates food for chewing and swallowing.

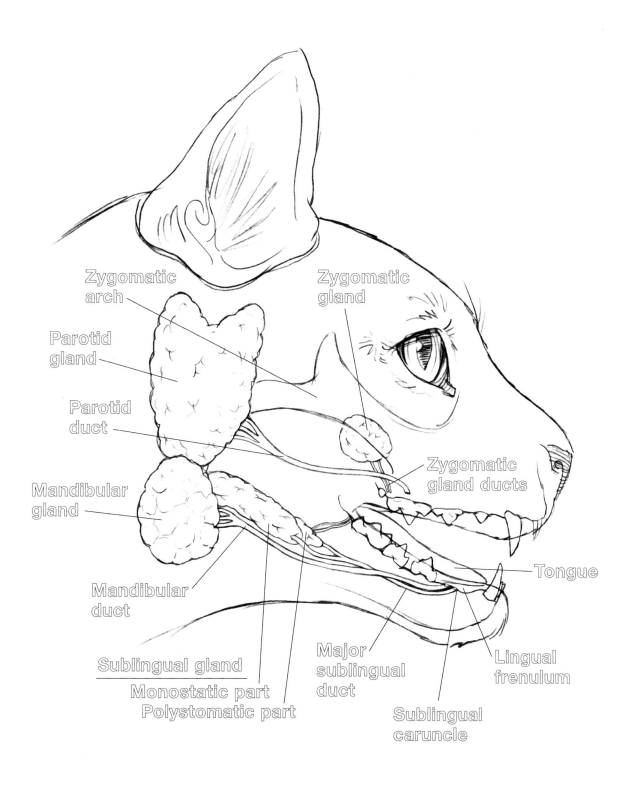

Zygomatic arch

Parotid gland

Parotid duct

Mandibular gland

Mandibular duct

Sublingual gland

Monostatic part
Polystomatic part

Zygomatic gland

Zygomatic gland ducts

Tongue

Major sublingual duct

Lingual frenulum

Sublingual caruncle

Oral Cavity, Tongue, Pharynx, and Esophagus

PLATE 46

Figure 1. Right lateral view of a sagittal section of a cat's head, nasal septum removed.
Figure 2. Dorsal view of the tongue and dissected laryngopharynx, trachea and esophagus.

Color each label in a different color and, where large enough, color the structure indicated.

The **pharynx** is a musculomembranous chamber common to the digestive and repiratory tracts. Its three parts are: 1) **Oropharynx** – ventral to the soft palate, 2) **nasopharynx** – dorsal to the soft palate, extending caudad from the choanae (exits from the nasal fossa on each side), 3) **laryngopharynx** - dorsal to the larynx and leading into the **esophagus**.

During swallowing, muscles raise the **tongue**, pressing food and water against the **hard palate**. The **soft palate** is elevated. The root of the tongue moves caudad and dorsad in a boltlike manner, pushing the **epiglottis** partially over the **laryngeal entrance**. The rima glottidis (space between the vocal folds) in the larynx is narrowed. Pressure by pharyngeal muscles forces food or water into the esophagus where automatic contractions carry food through to the stomach.

During breathing, the free edge of the soft palate is usually (but not always) under the epiglottis, and the laryngeal entrance is open.

Vallate, foliate and **fungiform papillae** contain taste buds, a complex of gustatory (taste) cells, supporting cells and nerve endings. Serous glands empty into the moat around a vallate papilla. **Conical, filiform** and **marginal papillae** do not contain taste buds. Marginal papillae occur along the edges of the nursing kitten's tongue.

Figure 1

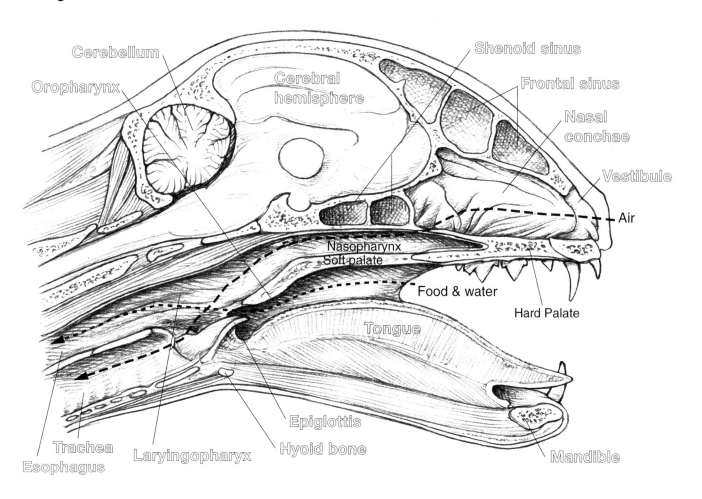

Cerebellum

Oropharynx

Cerebral hemisphere

Shenoid sinus

Frontal sinus

Nasal conchae

Vestibule

Air

Nasopharynx
Soft palate

Food & water

Hard Palate

Tongue

Epiglottis

Hyoid bone

Mandible

Trachea
Esophagus

Laryingopharyx

Figure 2

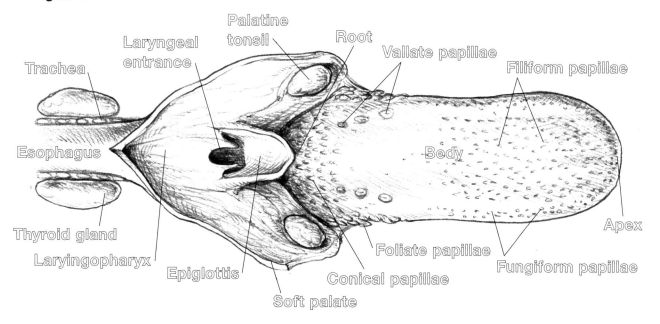

Trachea

Laryngeal entrance

Palatine tonsil

Root

Vallate papillae

Filiform papillae

Esophagus

Body

Thyroid gland

Apex

Laryingopharyx

Epiglottis

Soft palate

Conical papillae

Foliate papillae

Fungiform papillae

Contents of the Abdominal Cavity

PLATE 47

Figure 1. The abdominal wall and the thoracic muscles have been removed in this ventral view. The **greater omentum**, a double fold of peritoneum (serous membrane of the abdominal and pelvic cavities), enfolds the ventral and lateral aspects of the coils of the small intestine. A superficial leaf extends caudad from the surface of the stomach to near the urinary bladder, then turns back as a deep leaf that encloses the left limb of the pancreas and attaches to the dorsal part of the abdominal cavity. The collapsed cavity between the two leaves is called the omental bursa. It communicates with the main peritoneal cavity through a small opening, the epiploic foramen.

Notice the long deposits of fat (adipose tissue) that occur along small vessels in the greater omentum. Color the fat yellow. Use light red lines to indicate the rest of the greater omentum, which is transparent in life.

Minor parts of the greater omentum include an extension to the spleen, the gastrosplenic ligament, and a part that encloses some of the left lobe of the pancreas.

As a storage place for fat, large amounts accumulate in the greater omentum in obese cats. The greater omentum serves a protective function by the immune cells it contains. It assists injured tissues in forming new blood vessels. Once removed, the greater omentum does not regenerate.

Figure 2. The greater omentum has been removed, revealing the organs that it covered. Color the names and organs indicated.

Figure 1

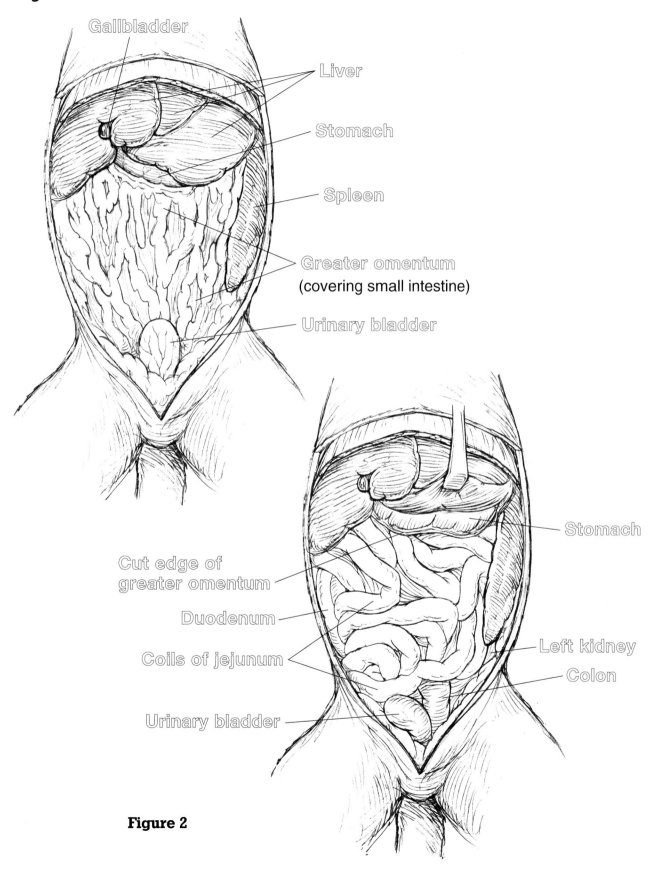

Gallbladder

Liver

Stomach

Spleen

Greater omentum
(covering small intestine)

Urinary bladder

Cut edge of
greater omentum

Duodenum

Coils of jejunum

Urinary bladder

Stomach

Left kidney

Colon

Figure 2

Stomach and Small Intestine

PLATE 48

Figure 1. Ventral view of feline stomach and small intestine (shortened).
Figure 2. Stomach and first part of the duodenum sectioned to expose the lining.

Using different colors, color the names, parts and regions indicated by the lines.

In Figure 1, The stomach is moderately full. Size and shape of the stomach vary greatly, depending on the amount of food (or gas) it contains. When empty, it does not touch the abdominal wall. Branches for the celiac artery course along the lesser and greater curvatures. Venous drainage is through branches of the portal vein to the liver.

Glands in the proper gastric gland region secrete hydrochloric acid and the enzymes pepsin (digests protein) and rennin (curdles milk). Superficial lining cells of the mucous membrane of the stomach secrete protective mucus.

The small intestine, suspended by the peritoneal mesentery, is approximately 3.5 times the length of the body. The bile duct (from the gall bladder) and the major pancreatic duct open on the major duodenal papilla; the minor pancreatic duct and the minor duodenal papilla are inconstant in the cat. The intestinal mucous membrane secretes enzymes and mucus. The mucous membrane lining the stomach and the small intestine also produce hormones. Peyer's patches, groups of lymphatic nodules, are prominent in the ileum. Branches from the cranial mesenteric artery supply most of the small intestine.

Inflammation of the lining of the stomach (gastritis) and the lining of the small intestine (enteritis) may be caused by different organisms or substances.

Vomiting is a natural function in cats. Hair balls that accumulate in the cat's stomach are frequently vomited.

Figure 1

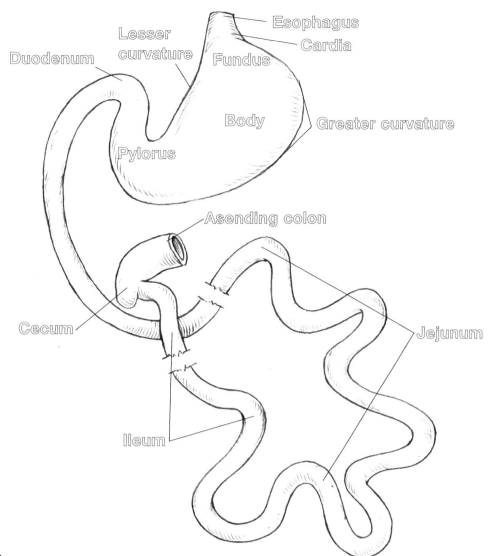

Figure 2

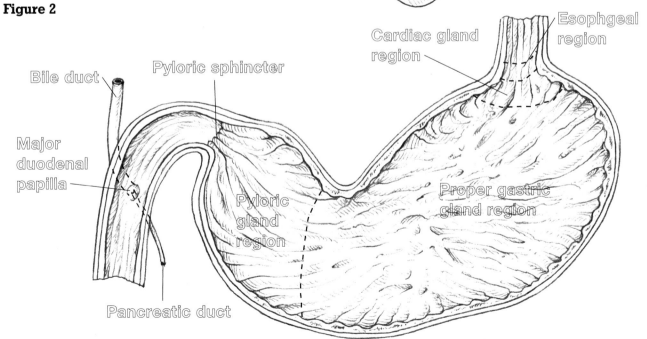

Liver and Pancreas

PLATE 49

Figure 1. Diaphragmatic surface of the feline liver.
Figure 2. Visceral surface of the feline liver.
Figure 3. Ventral view of the feline pancreas and related organs.

Color the names and the structures indicated, using different colors.

Peritoneum covers the liver, and four peritoneal ligaments stabilize the liver. The diaphragmatic surface is closely applied to the diaphragm; the visceral surface faces against the abdominal viscera (large internal organs). The stomach. left kidney and duodenum press firmly against the visceral surface.

Two blood vessels supply the liver:
1) The **portal vein** carries blood from the stomach, small intestine, part of the large intestine, pancreas and spleen to the liver's sinusoids, large capillaries between sheets of liver cells.
2) **Hepatic artery** branches supply nutrients, especially oxygen, to liver cells.

Branches of **hepatic veins** carry blood from the liver to the caudal vena cava. Blood brought to the liver contains absorbed nutrients and also harmful substances. The harmful substances are destroyed by the liver. Metabolic compounds are used to make many essential substances, including cholesterol and bile. Secreted bile is stored in the gall bladder and then transported by the bile duct to the duodenum. Here it helps to neutralize acid and emulsify fats, breaking up large fat globules into smaller ones.

The pancreas is two glands in one:
1) The exocrine part produces digestive enzymes that are carried to the duodenum by pancreatic duct. The accessory pancreatic duct is inconstant.
2) The endocrine part secretes the hormones, glucagon, insulin and somatostatin and pancreatic polypeptide into the blood for transport to tissues elsewhere in the body.

These homones are produced by specific cells in masses called pancreatic islets (islets of Langerhans), Glucagon mobilizes blood sugar from the liver; insulin decreases blood sugar; somatostatin inhibits the release of growth hormone from the pituitary gland and reduces contractions of smooth muscle in the intestines and gall bladder, pancreatic polypeptide inhibits exocrine pancreatic secretion.

Inflammation of the liver is termed hepatitis, a disease caused mainly by viruses, although other factors can cause hepatitis. (-itis = inflammation of.)

Inflammation of the pancreas is termed pancreatitis, a disease due to self digestion by its own enzymes. It may be caused by bile duct disease, increased fat in the blood or trauma (damage) to the abdomen.

Figure 1

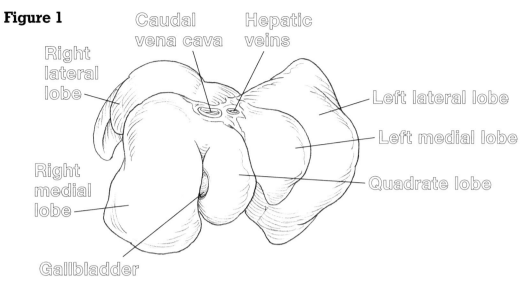

Caudal vena cava

Hepatic veins

Right lateral lobe

Left lateral lobe

Left medial lobe

Right medial lobe

Quadrate lobe

Gallbladder

Figure 2

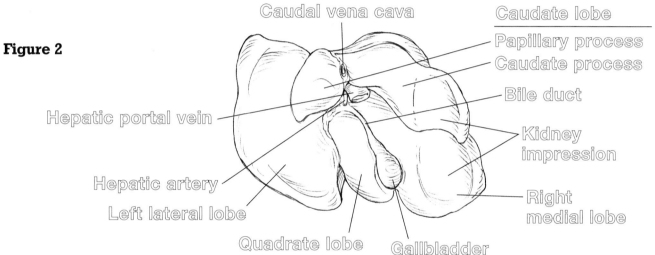

Caudal vena cava

Caudate lobe

Papillary process

Caudate process

Bile duct

Hepatic portal vein

Kidney impression

Hepatic artery

Left lateral lobe

Right medial lobe

Quadrate lobe

Gallbladder

Figure 3

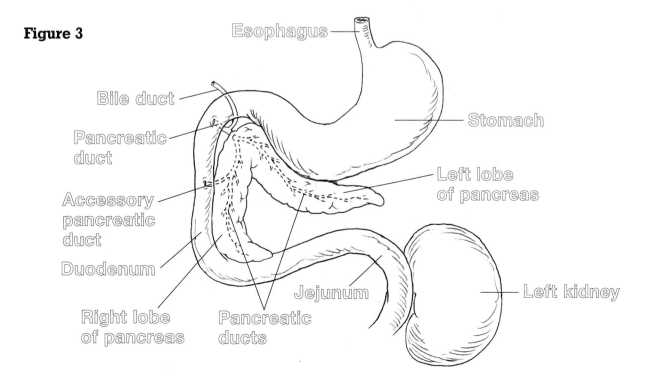

Esophagus

Bile duct

Stomach

Pancreatic duct

Accessory pancreatic duct

Left lobe of pancreas

Duodenum

Right lobe of pancreas

Pancreatic ducts

Jejunum

Left kidney

Large Intestine, Anus, and Anal Sacs

PLATE 50

Figure 1. Isolated large intestine.
Figure 2. Caudal view of the anus.
Figure 3. Dorsal view of sectioned rectum, anal canal and anal sacs.

Color the names and the organs and regions indicated.

The large intestine consists of the small **cecum**, the **colon** and **rectum**. The cecum and the **ileum** of the small intestine both empty into the **ascending colon**.

The primary functions of the large intestine are the absorption of water and a few other nutrients, production of mucus and formation of feces (stool). Like the stomach and small intestine, smooth muscle in the wall of the colon functions in <u>peristalsis</u>, the wave of contraction that moves the contents of these organs toward the anus.

Inflammation of the colon is termed <u>colitis</u>.

Each **anal sac** is actually a pouch of modified skin, opening by means of a duct on the **cutaneous zone** of the **anal canal**. The walls of an **anal sac** contain large oil (sebaceous) glands and modified sweat glands. The contents of the anal sacs consist of secretions of these glands and sloughed off cells from the lining epidermis. Normally, anal sacs are expressed by the passage of firm stool and from squeezing by the sphincter muscles on either side of each sac. Accumulation of anal sac secretion may be caused by prolonged soft stool or temporary plugging of the anal sac duct. An affected cat may scoot along on his/her rear because of discomfort. Manual expression of the contents may be necessary.

Circumanal glands extend from the skin into the subcutis superficial to the anal sacs. These strange glands contact sebaceous (oil) glands, but they lack ducts and do not appear to produce a secretion. Their function is unknown.

Figure 1

Figure 2

Figure 3

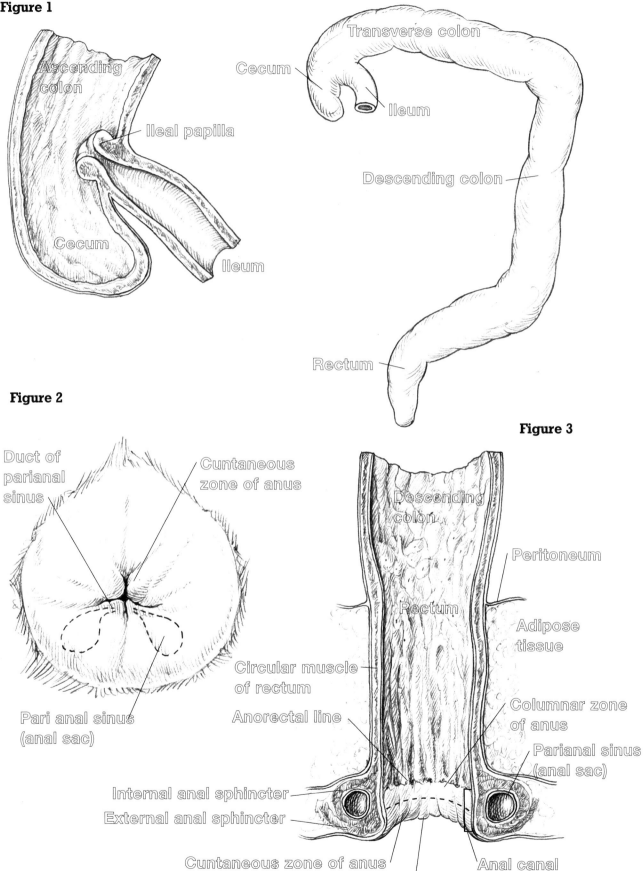

Ascending colon

Transverse colon

Cecum

Ileal papilla

Ileum

Cecum

Descending colon

Ileum

Rectum

Duct of parianal sinus

Cuntaneous zone of anus

Descending colon

Peritoneum

Rectum

Adipose tissue

Circular muscle of rectum

Pari anal sinus (anal sac)

Anorectal line

Columnar zone of anus

Parianal sinus (anal sac)

Internal anal sphincter

External anal sphincter

Cuntaneous zone of anus

Anal canal

Anus

Body Cavities and Serous Membranes

Thoracic, Abdominal and Pelvic Cavities

PLATE 51

Diagrammatic drawing of major body cavities lined by serous membranes of the female (queen). A serous membrane consists of a layer of mesothelium with subjacent loose connective tissue and a variable amount of white adipose tissue.

Peritoneum is divided into three continuous parts: Color the dashed lines without lifting your pencil from the paper.

1. **Parietal peritoneum** – lines abdominal cavity and part of pelvic cavity (L, paries = wall).

2. **Connecting peritoneum** – suspends organs by a double fold that encloses vessels and nerves.
   a. Mes + organ suspended: **mesentery** (G., mesos = middle + enteron = intestine)
   b. Peritoneal ligaments: suspend and support, e.g., **falciform ligament** of liver

3. **Visceral peritoneum** - encloses a viscus (L, large internal organ; pleural, viscera)

Peritoneum also suspends and encloses some of the male reproductive organs.

The musculomembranous diaphragm is covered by peritoneum on its abdominal surface; pleura on its thoracic surface.

Pleurae – two serous membranes, each continuous and forming a pleural sac.

1. **Parietal pleura** – lines each half of thoracic cavity: diaphragmatic pleura, costal pleura and mediastinal pleura. On each side, the mediastinal pleura limits the mediastinum, a space containing the heart, trachea, esophagus, the great blood vessels, nerves, thymus, loose connective tissue and adipose tissue.

2. **Visceral (pulmonary) pleura** – covers each lung.

Pericardium

1. Visceral serous pericardium – covers heart muscle and reflects around base of heart and great vessels

2. Parietal serous pericardium – covered by fibrous pericardium that blends with pericardial mediastinal pleura.

Serous cavities: peritoneal cavity, pleural cavity, pericardial cavity. Fine spaces between parietal and visceral serous membranes containing lubricating serous fluids (resembling blood serum).

Serous fluids increase in inflammatory conditions termed peritonitis, pleuritis and pericarditis.

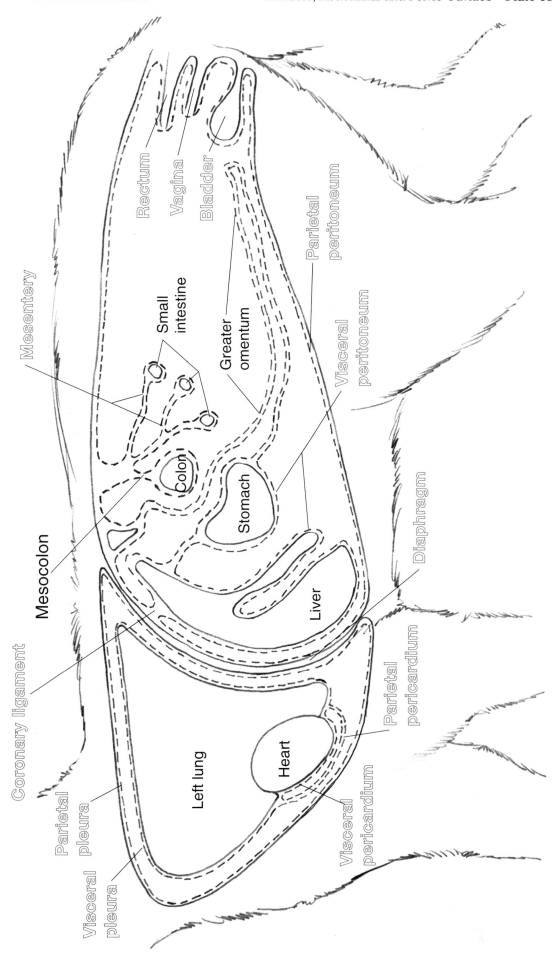

Rectum

Vagina

Bladder

Parietal peritoneum

Mesentery

Small intestine

Greater omentum

Visceral peritoneum

Colon

Stomach

Mesocolon

Liver

Diaphragm

Coronary ligament

Parietal pericardium

Left lung

Heart

Parietal pleura

Visceral pericardium

Visceral pleura

In Place Positions of Internal Organs

PLATE 52

Figure 1. Right lateral view of the internal organs of the female (queen).
Figure 2. Left lateral view of the internal organs of the male (stud).

Color the names and the organs indicated.

Relations of organs to each other and to the exterior of the body are important in the following procedures:
1. Palpation – feeling from the exterior or through an organ that opens to the exterior, for example, the rectum.
2. Auscultation – listening to normal and abnormal sounds from internal organs, mainly the lungs, heart, arteries, stomach and intestines. A stethoscope is a device used to convey these sounds to one's ears.
3. Percussion – striking short, sharp blows on a region and listening for sounds obtained from underlying organs.
4. Surgical approaches to internal organs. A knowledge of these relations is essential for determining where to make incisions.
5. Interpretation of radiographic and ultrasonic images.

Figure 1

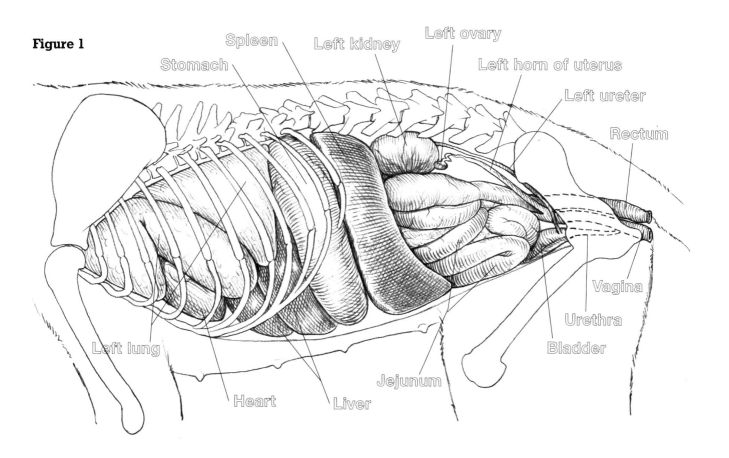

Spleen

Stomach

Left kidney

Left ovary

Left horn of uterus

Left ureter

Rectum

Left lung

Heart

Liver

Jejunum

Vagina

Urethra

Bladder

Figure 2

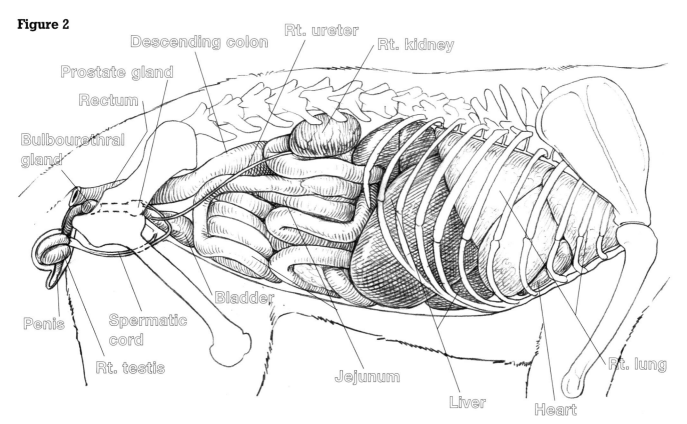

Descending colon

Rt. ureter

Rt. kidney

Prostate gland

Rectum

Bulbourethral gland

Penis

Rt. testis

Spermatic cord

Bladder

Jejunum

Liver

Heart

Rt. lung

Cardiovascular System

Major Circulatory Patterns

PLATE 53

Color the names of organs and regions.

Coloring the arrows blue, trace the flow of poorly-oxygenated blood:

From the **cranial** and **caudal caval veins** (L., venae cavae) to the **right atrium**

Through the **right atrioventricular valve** to the **right ventricle**

Out of the heart through the **pulmonary valve** into the pulmonary circulation

Through the **pulmonary trunk** and **left and right pulmonary arteries** to the lungs

Finally, to capillaries (smallest blood vessels) in the walls of alveoli (little air sacs) in the lungs.

Here carbon dioxide is released from hemoglobin in erythrocytes (red blood cells) and oxygen is bound to the hemoglobin and is in the plasma for transport to the body's tissues.

Coloring the arrows red, trace the flow of oxygenated blood. Underline the names of organs and regions.

From capillaries in the lungs, through **pulmonary veins** to the **left atrium**

Through the **left atrioventricular valve** to the **left ventricle**

Then through the **aortic valve** into the **aorta** and the systemic circulation.

Color the arrows in arteries red; arrows in veins, blue. Satellite (companion) veins accompany most arteries In the hepatic portal system, blood in veins coming from the stomach, pancreas, spleen and intestines is carried by the **portal vein** to sinusoidal capillaries in the liver. From these capillaries, blood is carried by **hepatic veins** to the **caudal caval vein** (L., vena cava caudalis) Color veins blue.

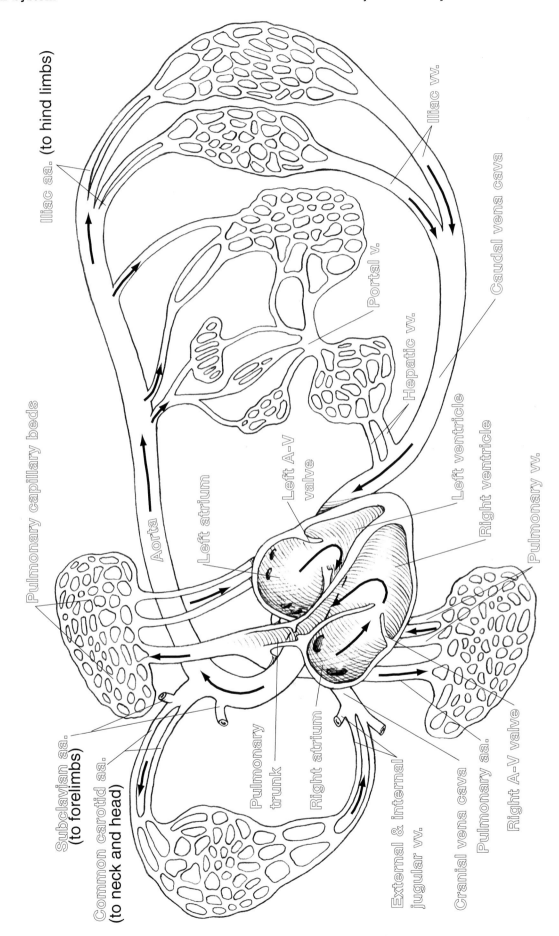

Iliac aa. (to hind limbs)

Iliac vv.

Caudal vena cava

Portal v.

Hepatic vv.

Pulmonary capillary beds

Aorta

Left atrium

Left A-V valve

Left ventricle

Right ventricle

Pulmonary vv.

Subclavian aa. (to forelimbs)

Common carotid aa. (to neck and head)

Pulmonary trunk

Right atrium

External & internal jugular vv.

Cranial vena cava

Pulmonary aa.

Right A-V valve

The Feline Heart

PLATE 54

Figure 1. Left lateral view of isolated heart and great vessels. Coronary arteries are the first branches of the aorta. **Auricles** are outpocketings of **atria**. Color the names and structures indicated in these drawings.

Figure 2. Sectioned heart, exposing its chambers. A cardiac skeleton of fibrous tissue and some cartilage separates the cardiac muscle of the atria from that of the ventricles. A-V = atrioventricular

The **arterial ligament** is a remnant of the arterial duct (L., ductus arteriosus) that shunted blood from the pulmonary trunk to the aorta in the fetus (unborn kitten) An oval foramen carried blood from the right atrium to the left atrium in the fetal heart. Most of the blood flowing into the fetal heart is shunted through these two passages, bypassing the pulmonary circulation. Since the fetal lungs are not functioning, mother's blood in the placenta supplies oxygen to the fetus.

During beating of the heart, the two atria fill and contract. Then the two ventricles fill and contract, forcing blood into the pulmonary trunk and the aorta.

Heart sounds are caused by the rush of blood and the closing heart valves, first the A-V valves, then the pulmonary and aortic semilunar valves. The **sinoatrial node** in the wall of the right atrium is the pacemaker (controlled by the nervous system) that begins the rhythmic contractions of the atria. Cardiac muscle fibers conduct impulses to the atrioventricular node in the wall (septum) between the atria. Specialized cardiac muscle fibers (Purkinje fibers) descend from the atrioventricular node, through the cardiac skeleton to each side of the interventricular septum, branching to supply the ventricles, and causing their contraction. A moderator band extends from the interventricular septum to the lateral wall of the right ventricle.

Heart disease, mostly relating to endocarditis and a dilatation (abnormal dilation) of the heart resulting in a weak, rapid pulse, is fairly common in cats. Another type of cardiomyopathy occurs when the heart walls becomes thickened and over-developed this is called hypertrophic cardiomyopathy. Cardiac dysfunction is often a result of another problem, such as hyperthyroidism, that stresses the heart. Infections can cause heart trouble. Long-term congenital defects of the heart can gradually weaken the heart as it attempts to compensate for the defect.

Figure 1

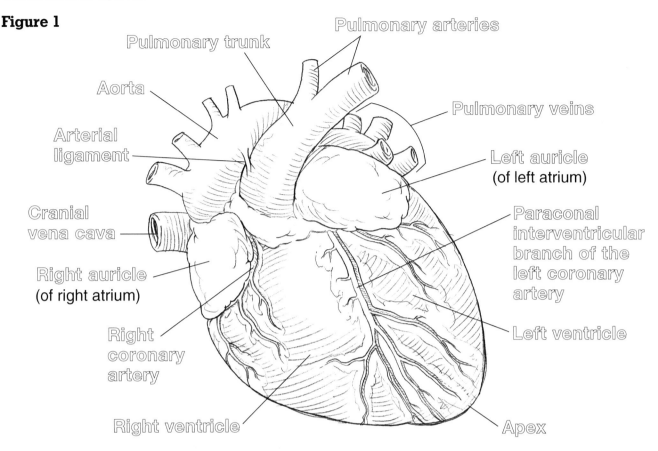

Pulmonary trunk

Pulmonary arteries

Aorta

Pulmonary veins

Arterial
ligament

Left auricle
(of left atrium)

Cranial
vena cava

Paraconal
interventricular
branch of the
left coronary
artery

Right auricle
(of right atrium)

Left ventricle

Right
coronary
artery

Right ventricle

Apex

Figure 2

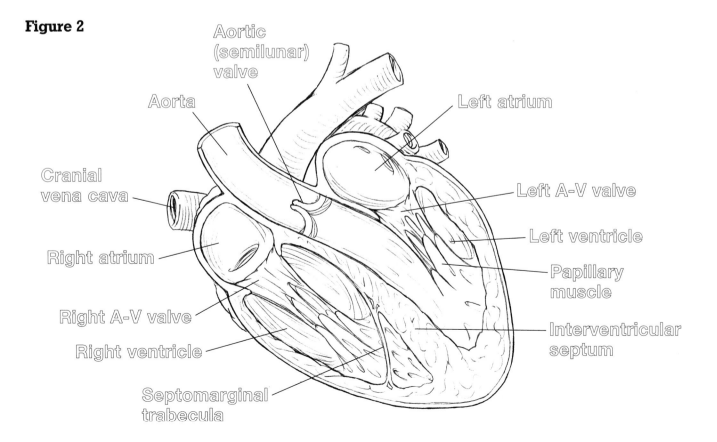

Aortic
(semilunar)
valve

Aorta

Left atrium

Cranial
vena cava

Left A-V valve

Right atrium

Left ventricle

Papillary
muscle

Right A-V valve

Interventricular
septum

Right ventricle

Septomarginal
trabecula

Vessels and Related Organs in the Thoracic Cavity

PLATE 55

Underline the boldfaced names in different colors and color indicated organs on the drawings. Color arteries red, veins blue and nerves yellow. Satellite veins not seen here.

Figure 1. Dissected thorax of a cat opened from left side.

1. **Aorta**
2. **L. vagus nerve**
3. **L. subclavian artery**
4. **L. costocervical trunk**
5. **L. vertebral a.**
6. **L. internal thoracic a.**
7. **L. superficial cervical a.**
8. **L. axillary a.**
9. **Brachiocephalic trunk**
10. **L. common carotid a.**
11. **Pulmonary trunk**
12. **L. pulmonary a.**
13. **Cranial vena cava**
14. **L. intercostal aa.**
15. **Pulmonary veins**
16. **Caudal vena cava**
17. **L. phrenic n. (to diaphragm)**
18. **Thoracic duct**
19. **Rt. Common cartotid**
20. **Rt. Subclavian**

Figure 2. Dissected thorax of a cat opened from right side.

1. **Aorta**
2. **Caudal vena cava**
3. **R. vagus nerve**
4. **Azygous vein**
5. **Cranial vena cava**
6. **Brachiocephalic trunk**
7. **R. vertebral a**
8. **R. costocervical trunk**
9. **R. common carotid a.**
10. **R. subclavian a.**
11. **R. internal thoracic a.**
12. **R. superficial cervical a.**
13. **R. axillary a.**
14. **R. phrenic n.**
15. **Internal thoracic v.**
16. **R. brachiocephalic v.**
17. **L. brachiocephalic v.**

Three passages perforate the **diaphragm**, the musculomembranous partition between the thoracic and abdominal cavities:

Ah. Aortic hiatus – transmits aorta, azygous vein and chyle cistern (beginning of thoracic duct).
Eh. Esophageal hiatus – transmits esophagus and vagus nerves
Fvc. Vena caval foramen (foramen venae cavae) – transmits caudal caval vein.

Figure 1

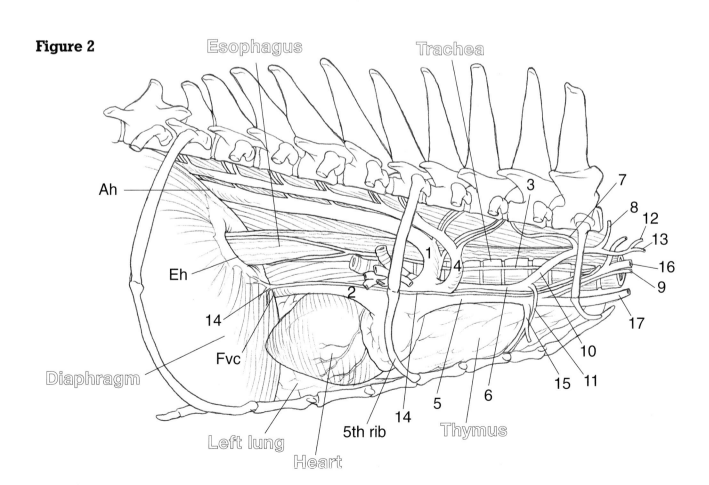

Figure 2

Vessels of the Abdominal Cavity

PLATE 56

Ventral view. Underline the **boldfaced names** of the vessels. Color arteries (a.) red, veins (v.) blue on the drawings.

Figure 1. Branches of aorta:

1. Celiac a.
2. L. gastric a.
3. Esophageal a.
4. Hepatic a.
5. Branches to liver
6. R. gastric a.
7. R. gastroepiploic a.
8. Cranial pancreaticoduodenal a.
9. Splenic a.
10. Branches to pancreas
11. Branches to spleen

12. L. gastroepiploic a.
13. Cranial mesenteric a.
14. Ileocolic a.
15. Middle colic a.
16. R. colic a.
17. Ileal a.
18. Caudal pancreaticoduodenal a.
19. Jejunal aa.
20. L. phenicoabdominal a.
21. L. renal a.
22. L. ovarian a.

(testicular a.)
23. Caudal mesenteric a.
24. Cranial rectal a.
25. L. colic a.

Branches of caudal caval vein:
26. Hepatic vv.
27. L. phrenicoabdominal v.
28. L. renal v.
29. L. ovarian vein
(L. testicular v.)
30. R. ovarian v.

Figure 2. Branches of portal vein:

31. Gastroduodenal v.
32. R. gastric v.
33. R. gastroepiploic v.
34. Cranial pancreaticoduodenal v.
35. Splenic v.
36. L. gastric v.
37. L. gastroepiploic v.

38. Branches from spleen
39. Branch from pancreas
40. Ileocolic v.
41. R. colic v.
42. Cranial mesenteric v.
43. Caudal pancreaticoduodenal v.
43.a Doudenal branches

44. Jejunal vv.
45. Caudal mesenteric v.
46. Middle colic v.
47. L. colic v.

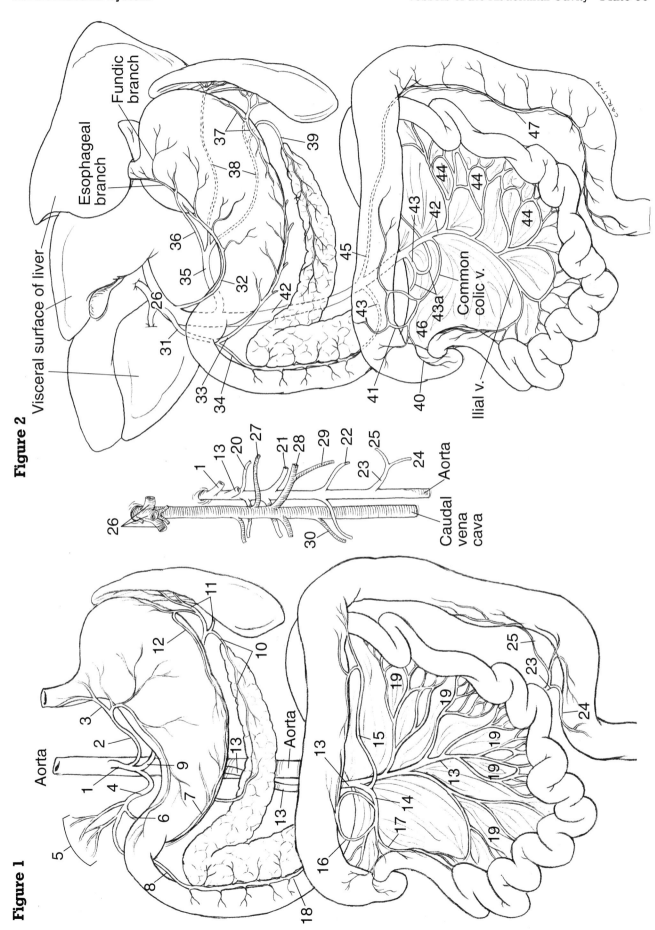

Figure 2

Esophageal branch

Fundic branch

Visceral surface of liver

37
38
39
36
35
32
42
43
45
44
44
44
44
47
43
42
43a
46
Common colic v.
41
40
Ilial v.
31
26
33
34

Figure 1

Aorta
1
13
20
27
21
28
29
22
23
25
24
Aorta
Caudal vena cava
26
30

Aorta
3
2
1
4
9
7
6
5
8
10
11
12
13
13
Aorta
13
15
19
19
19
19
19
19
19
13
14
17
16
18
25
23
24

CARLSON

Superficial Vessels of the Head and Neck

PLATE 57

Figure 1. Superficial and deep arteries. Right lateral view.
Figure 2. Superficial and deep veins. Right lateral view.

Underline the **boldfaced names** and color each artery (a.) red, each vein(v.) blue.

ARTERIES
1. **Common carotid a.**
2. **Cranial thyroid a.**
3. **Internal carotid a.**
4. **External carotid a.**
5. **Cranial laryngeal a.**
6. **Occipital a.**
7. **Ascending pharyngeal a.**
8. **Lingual a.**
9. **Facial a.**
10. **Caudal auricular a.**
11. **Superficial temporal a.**
12. **Transverse facial a.**
13. **Lat. dorsal palpebral a.**
14. **Lat. ventral palpebral a.**
15. **Maxillary a.**
16. **Infraorbital a.**
17. **Nasal aa.**

VEINS
18. **External jugular v.**
19. **Linguofacial v.**
20. **Lingual vein**
21. **Hyoid venous arch**
22. **Sublingual v.**
23. **Facial v.**
24. **Inferior labial v.**
25. **Deep facial v.**
26. **Superior labial v.**
27. **Nasal vv.**
28. **Angular ocular v.**
29. **Ophthalmic v.**
30. **Maxillary v.**
31. **Great auricular v.**
32. **Superior temporal v.**
33. **Pterygoid plexus**

Figure 1

Figure 2

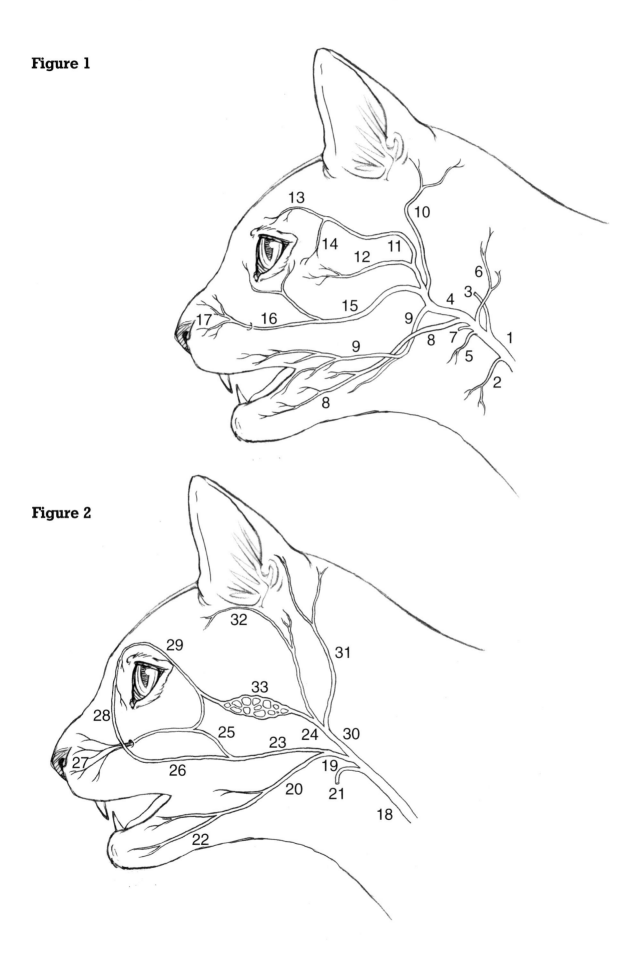

The Feline Pulse and Venipuncture Sites

PLATE 58

Figure 1.

A. Taking the cat's pulse by palpating the **femoral artery** just deep to the skin and fascia in the femoral triangle on the medial aspect of the upper thigh. The hand is wrapped around the cranial aspect of the thigh.

B. Skin and fascia removed from the medial aspect of the left thigh, exposing the femoral triangle, a space between the caudal belly of the **sartorial m.** cranially and the **pectineal m.** caudally. Fingertips are superimposed over the femoral a.

Figure 2. A cat lying on the right side with the left elbow moved craniad. The heartbeat may be felt (or auscultated) in the fifth and sixth intercostal spaces just dorsal to the sternum.

Figure 3. Site for venipuncture of the **medial saphenous vein.**

Figure 4. Site for venipuncture of the **cephalic vein.** Color the names and the structures indicated, coloring the femoral artery and the heart red, veins blue and muscles pink.

The pulse is the rhythmic expansion of an artery that may be felt with the fingers. The pulse rate reflects the heart rate – the number of heart beats per minute. The normal resting heart rate of cats varies between 120 and 200 beats per minute. The heart beat may be felt in cats by grasping around the sternum with the thumb on one side and fingers on the opposite side where the elevated elbow will touch the chest. The femoral artery is palpable just distal to the femoral triangle. The femoral pulse is easier to assess and more accurate than assessing the heartbeat.

Tachycardia is the term for an excessively rapid heart beat. Bradycardia is an abnormal slowing of the heart beat. An abnormal sound coming from the heart is termed a murmur. It

may be an "innocent murmur", or it may indicate an abnormal condition of the heart.

The veins at the venipuncture sites lie immediately deep to the skin, subcutis and fascia. Small branches of the medial cutaneous antebrachial nerve parallel the cephalic vein. Sensation to the lateral skin of the leg is provided by branches from the superficial peroneal and lateral cutaneous sural nerves. Compression of a vein proximal to the site of venipuncture, distends the vein and makes it easier to insert a needle or catheter (long plastic tube). Compression is released for injection. The femoral vein may be used for venipuncture without compression proximal to the needle.

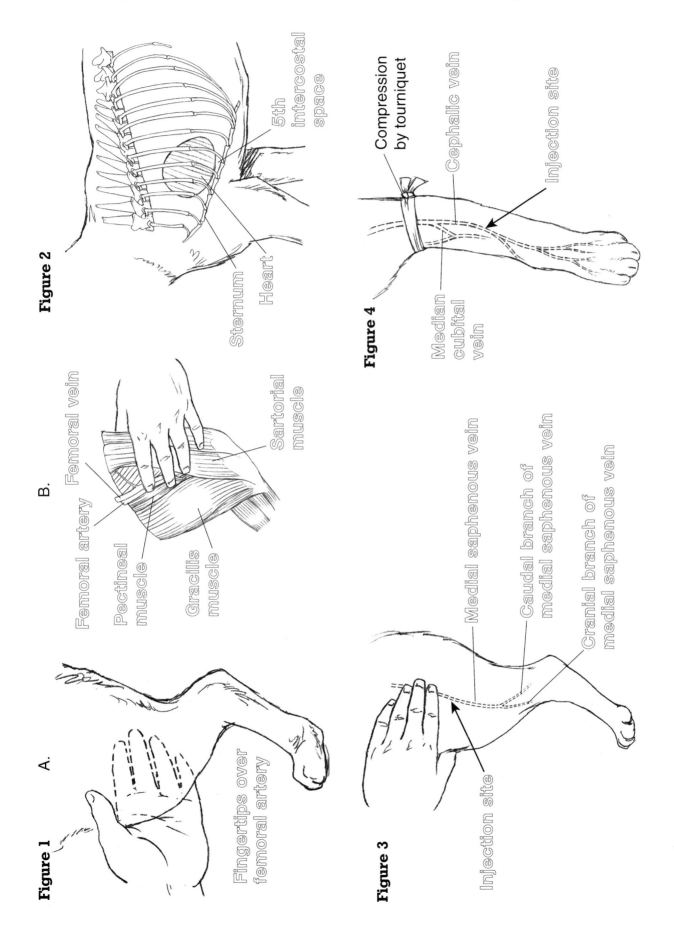

Figure 2

5th intercostal space

Sternum

Heart

Figure 4

Compression by tourniquet

Cephalic vein

Injection site

Median cubital vein

B.

Femoral vein

Sartorial muscle

Femoral artery

Pectineal muscle

Gracillis muscle

Figure 1

A.

Fingertips over femoral artery

Figure 3

Medial saphenous vein

Caudal branch of medial saphenous vein

Cranial branch of medial saphenous vein

Injection site

Immune System

Bone Marrow, Thymus, and Spleen

PLATE 59

Organs of the immune system produce cells and their products that combat bacteria, viruses and cancer cells.

Color the names and the drawings of these organs indicated on the drawing.

Red bone marrow produces red blood cells (erythrocytes), white blood cells (leukocytes -- neutrophils, eosinophils, basophils, B and T lymphocytes, monocytes) and platelets. Platelets are fragments of large cells (megakarocytes) in bone marrow that are essential for blood clotting. Red marrow occupies spaces in spongy bone in long bones, vertebrae, ribs, sternebrae and flat bones. Sternebrae and the wing of the ilium are sites for obtaining bone marrow samples.

Yellow bone marrow in the medullary cavity consists primarily of fat cells, but blood-cell-producing units of stem cells can begin to generate blood cells again in some cases of anemia (lack of quality or quantity of red blood cells). Production of abnormal leukocytes is termed leukemia.

The **thymus** continues to grow until puberty, occupying the cranial part of the mediastinum and extending through the thoracic inlet into the neck next to the trachea. Then it gradually becomes smaller (involutes), persisting as a small organ in the cranial part of the mediastinum in the adult. The thymus produces white blood cells called T-cell lymphocytes. These cells populate the spleen, lymph nodes and bone marrow.

Since it is attached to the stomach by the greater omentum, the position of the **spleen** in the left side of the abdominal cavity changes slightly as the stomach changes shape or the spleen swells with blood. The capsule and trabeculae (little beams) of the feline spleen contain smooth muscle that contracts to move stored blood into the circulation. Other functions of the spleen include: 1. Formation of red blood cells in the fetus; 2. Destruction of old red blood cells and particles in the blood; 3. Production of lymphocytes in the white pulp.

The spleen is not essential to life, and it may be removed surgically if it grows abnormally large or if it ruptures.

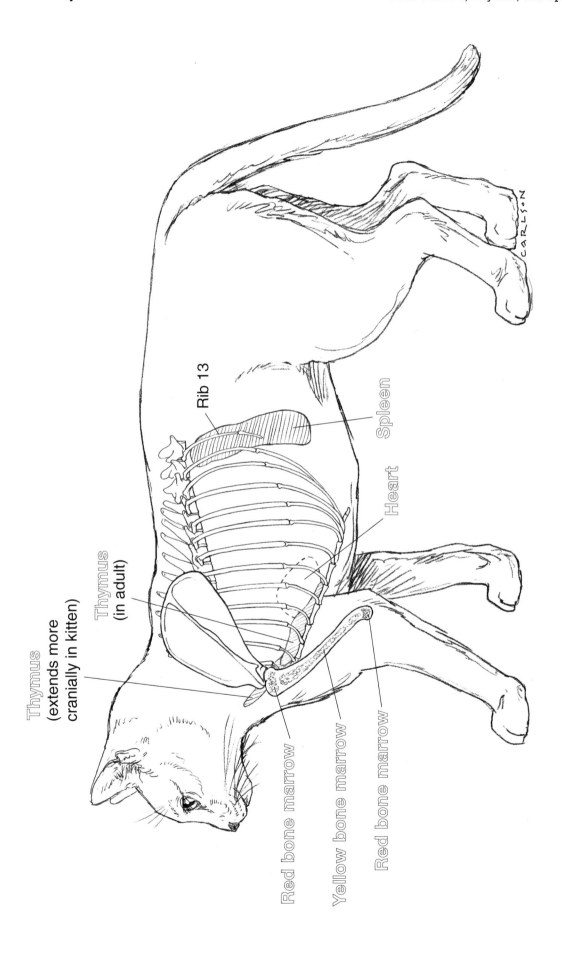

Rib 13

Spleen

Heart

Thymus
(in adult)

Thymus
(extends more
cranially in kitten)

Red bone marrow

Yellow bone marrow

Red bone marrow

Lymph Nodes and Lymph Vessels

PLATE 60

A **lymphocenter (lc.)** is a **lymph node (ln.)** or a group of lymph nodes that receive lymphatic (lymph) vessels draining a given region of the body. A fraction of tissue fluid that is not returned to blood capillaries is moved by tissue turgor pressure that forces it into lymph capillaries and then into larger lymphatics. Lymph within these vessels filters through a series of lymph nodes and connecting lymph vessels that eventually return lymph to the large veins. Phagocytes (cell-eating cells) in lymph nodes remove foreign particles, bacteria and cancer cells from lymph. Lymph nodes also produce lymphocytes.

Underline the names and color the lymphocenters (lc) and lymph vessels on the drawing. Arrows indicate lymph flow.

1. **Parotid lc.** – one ln.
2. **Mandibular lc.** – 2 lnn.
3. **Retropharyngeal lc.** – medial ln larger than lateral ln
4. **Deep cervical lc.**
   Cranial, middle and caudal cervical lnn.
5. **Left tracheal trunk**
6. **Superficial cervical lc.**
7. **Right lymphatic trunk**
8. **Dorsal thoracic lc.**
9. **Thoracic duct** – Empties into cranial caval vein
10. **Bronchial lc.** – Tracheobronchial lnn., pulmonary lnn
11. **Mediastinal lc.** – Cranial, middle and caudal
    mediastinal lnn.
12. **Ventral thoracic lc.** – Sternal lnn.
13. **Axillary lc.** – Axillary & accessory axillary lnn.
14. **Chyle cistern** – Receives lymphatic trunks
    Origin of thoracic duct
15. **Celiac lc.** – Hepatic lnn., gastric lnn., splenic lnn.,
    pancreaticoduodenal lnn.
16. **Cranial mesenteric lc.** – Jejunal lnn., Right, middle and
    left colic lnn.
17. **Lumbar lc.** – Lumbar aortic lnn., renal lnn.
18. **Lumbar trunks**
19. **Intestinal trunks**
20. **Iliosacral lc.** – Medial iliac lnn., sacral lnn.
    hypogastric lnn.,
21. **Iliofemoral lc.**
    Iliofemoral ln. femoral ln. – small and inconstant
22. **Superficial inguinal lc.**
    Scrotal lnn in male. Mammary lnn.in female
23. **Popliteal lc.** – one large ln.

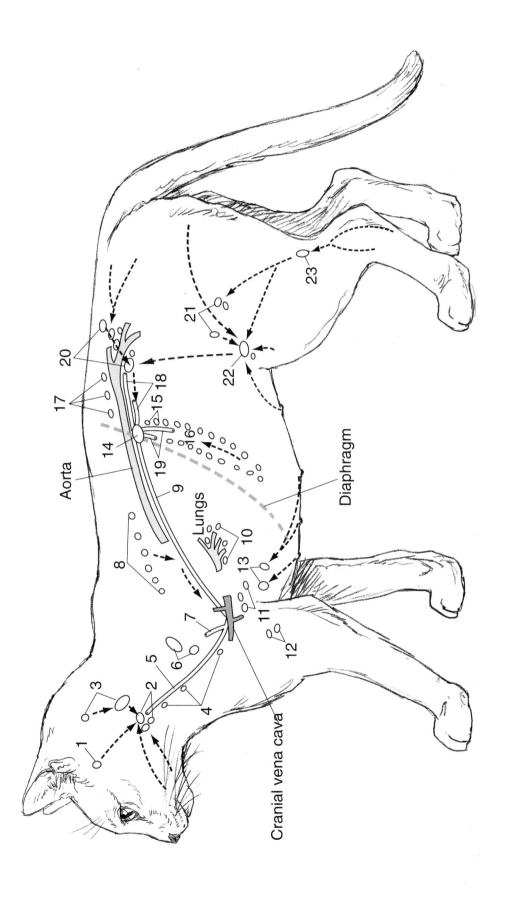

Aorta

Diaphragm

Lungs

Cranial vena cava

1
2
3
4
5
6
7
8
9
10
11
12
13
14
15
16
17
18
19
20
21
22
23

Tonsils

PLATE 61

In this drawing, the root of the tongue is depressed to visualize the **palatine tonsils**, each slightly protruding from a <u>tonsillar sinus</u>.

Color the names and the structures indicated.

A tonsil is a small mass of lymphoid tissue under the mucous membrane. Efferent lymphatic vessels carry lymph and lymphocytes from tonsils.

The cat has three pairs of tonsils:
1. **Palatine tonsils** – in the lateral walls of the oropharynx.
2. <u>Pharyngeal tonsils</u> (adenoids) - lymphatic nodules in the nasopharynx. (Not seen here.)
3. <u>Lingual tonsils</u> – diffuse in the base of the tongue. Not visible grossly.

When the palatine tonsils are inflamed (<u>tonsillitis</u>), greatly enlarged and painful, the cat has difficulty swallowing and eating.

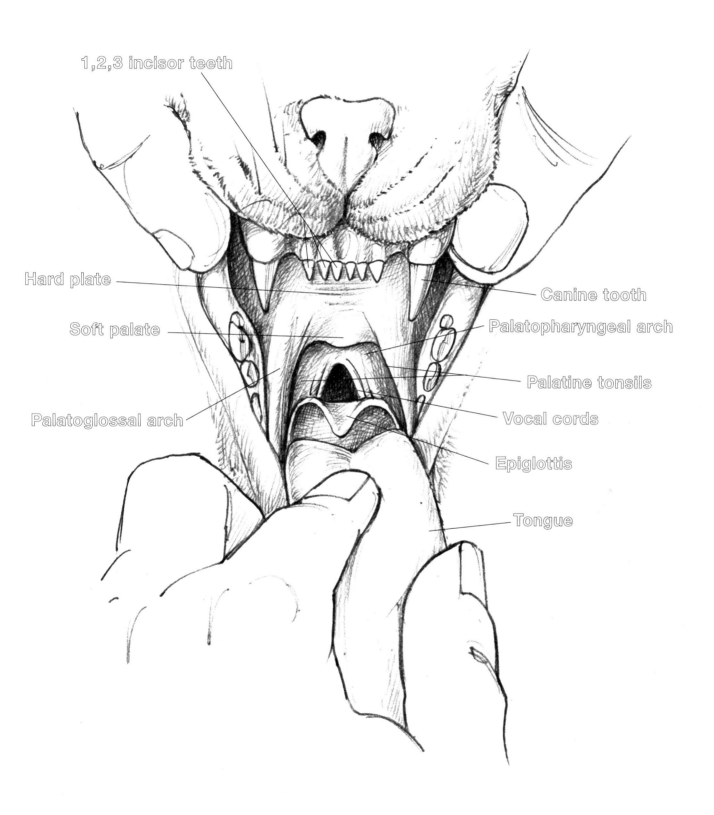

1,2,3 incisor teeth

Hard plate

Soft palate

Palatoglossal arch

Canine tooth

Palatopharyngeal arch

Palatine tonsils

Vocal cords

Epiglottis

Tongue

Respiratory System

Nasal Cavity and Nasopharynx

PLATE 62

Figure 1. Sagittal section of the cat's head with the nasal septum removed, revealing the interior of the left nasal fossa (half of the nasal cavity).

Color the names on the drawings and the structures indicated.

A short arrow indicates the entrance to the <u>auditory tube</u> that connects with the tympanic cavity of the middle ear, admitting air into the middle ear. This anatomic arrangement serves to equalize air pressure on each side of the eardrum.

Color the names and structures indicated.

There are three pharynges (plural of pharynx): 1. **Oropharynx** ventral to the soft palate, 2. **nasopharynx** dorsal to the soft palate, extending caudad from the choanae (exits from the nasal fossa on each side), 3. **laryngopharynx** around the larynx and leading into the esophagus.

In this drawing, the soft palate is in the breathing position, directing air into the larynx.

An abnormality, <u>dorsal displacement of the soft palate</u>, prevents the soft palate from returning to the normal breathing position after swallowing has occurred. Surgical correction is indicated.

Figure 2. Shows the course of the duct of lateral nasal gland and the course of the **nasolacrimal duct** carrying tears from the conjunctival sac in front of the eye.

Figure 1

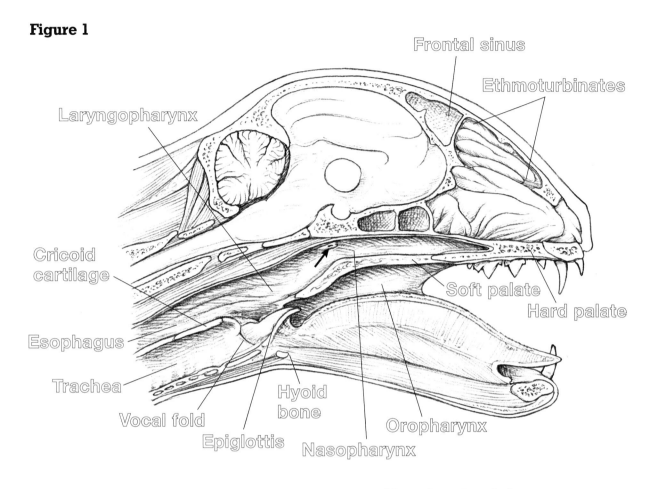

Frontal sinus

Ethmoturbinates

Laryngopharynx

Cricoid cartilage

Esophagus

Trachea

Vocal fold

Hyoid bone

Epiglottis

Nasopharynx

Oropharynx

Soft palate

Hard palate

Figure 2

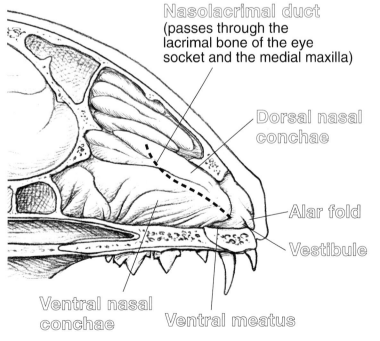

Nasolacrimal duct
(passes through the
lacrimal bone of the eye
socket and the medial maxilla)

Dorsal nasal conchae

Alar fold

Vestibule

Ventral nasal conchae

Ventral meatus

Larynx

PLATE 63

Figure 1. Right lateral view of laryngeal cartilages and cranial tracheal rings.
Figure 2. Dorsal view of larynx. Pharynx and esophagus cut mid-dorsally.
Figure 3. Right lateral view of laryngeal muscles. Right half of thyroid cartilage; thyroarytenoid muscle and most of cricothyroid muscle removed.
Figure 4. Median section of the larynx. A dashed line indicates extent of the laryngeal ventricle. Three regions of the laryngeal cavity are: **A. vestibule, B. glottis** and **C. infraglottic cavity**

Underline the **boldfaced names** and color indicated structures on the drawings.

1. **Hyoid bones**
2. **Epiglottic cartilage**
3. **Hyoepglottic m.**
4. **Thyroid cartilage**
5. **Cricoid cartilage**
6. **Trachea, tracheal rings**
7. **Cricothyroid ligament**
8. **Thyrohyoid ligament**
9. **Processes of arytenoid cartilage**
10. **Transverse arytenoid m.**
11. **Dorsal cricoarytenoid m.**
12. **Lateral cricoarytenoid m.**
13. **Vocal m.**
14. **Vocal ligament**
15. **Vestibular m.**
16. **Vestibular fold**
17. **Vocal fold**
18. **Aryepiglottic fold**

All of the intrinsic muscles of the larynx except the cricothyroid muscles receive their motor supply from the caudal laryngeal nerves.

Functions of the larynx:
1. Regulates the volume of air passing through in inspiration and expiration.
2. Prevents foreign material from entering the trachea through partial closure by the epiglottis and constriction of the glottis.
3. Phonation (vocalization) – caused by variations in air flow, vibrations of vocal folds and air in laryngeal ventricles.

Figure 1

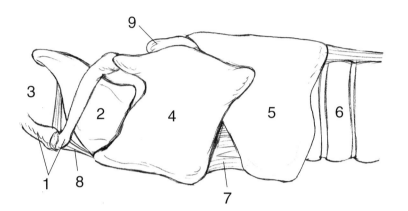

Figure 2

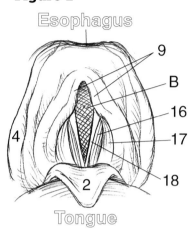

Figure 3

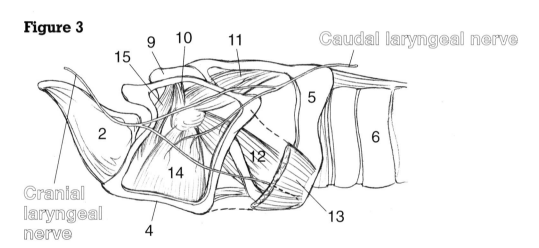

Figure 4

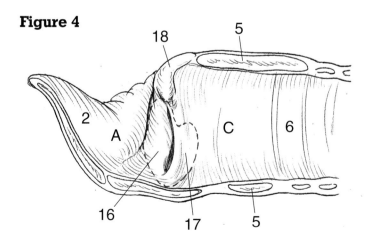

Trachea and Lungs

PLATE 64

Figure 1. Ventral view of **trachea** and **lungs**. Lobes of lungs separated. Diagrammatic drawing of **bronchial tree**.
Figure 2. Cross section of a **tracheal ring**.
Figure 3. Microscopic view of **alveoli** (L., little hollows), tiny air sacs with capillaries in their walls.

Color the names and the structures indicated on the drawings.

The trachea extends from the cricoid cartilage through the neck into the mediastinum to the bifurcation (fork) dorsal to the base of the heart. It consists of around 38 to 43 incomplete C-shaped rings of cartilage. Dorsally, the open part of each ring is closed by smooth muscle, the **tracheal muscle**, and fibrous connective tissue. Longitudinal ligaments of fibroelastic connective tissue connect the rings. This tissue continues under the mucous membrane of the two **principal bronchi**, gradually becoming thinner in the smaller conducting airways.

Where the trachea bifurcates into **left** and **right principal bronchi**, gaps in the free ends of the tracheal rings are filled by plates of cartilage. Cartilaginous plates continue on to support the walls of the bronchi (singular – bronchus) They are not present in the smallest airways, the bronchioles. Smooth muscle in the walls of airways serve to constrict them. Glands and cells in the mucous membrane produce mucous and serous secretions. Beginning with the nasal cavity, cilia on the cells lining the airways move secretions toward the exterior.

A final **terminal bronchiole** (which has ciliated cells but lacks mucus-secreting cells) leads to alveolar ducts that, in turn, give off alveoli. Gas exchange of carbon dioxide from red blood cells and oxygen into them takes place between air within alveoli and blood within capillaries in alveolar walls.

The normal breathing rate of cats varies with their size. The rate may be affected by excitement, exercise, age, illness, environmental temperature, pregnancy and a full digestive tract. Rapid breathing serves to cool the body by increased dead-space ventilation -- the volume of air that does not take part in gas exchange over a given period. The increased movement of air evaporates secretions in the oral cavity, helping to cool the body. This compensates for the lack of liquid sweat on feline skin. Panting - rapid breathing with the mouth open and often with the tongue protracted - is uncommon in cats. It is associated with atmospheric heat, stress and exercise or in diseased states of the respiratory or cardiovascular systems.

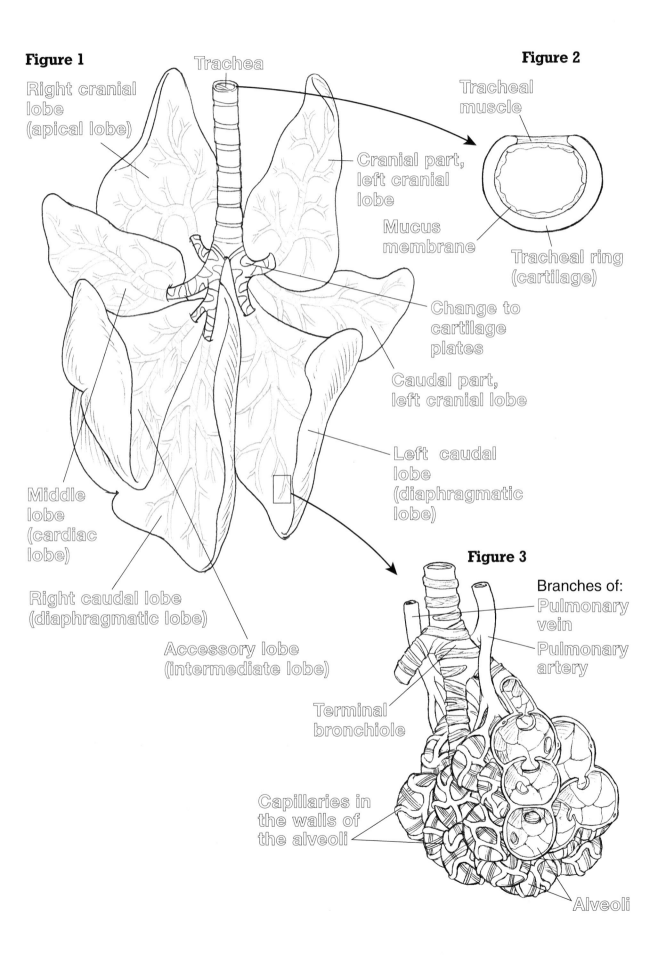

Figure 1

Right cranial lobe (apical lobe)

Trachea

Figure 2

Tracheal muscle

Cranial part, left cranial lobe

Mucus membrane

Tracheal ring (cartilage)

Change to cartilage plates

Caudal part, left cranial lobe

Left caudal lobe (diaphragmatic lobe)

Middle lobe (cardiac lobe)

Right caudal lobe (diaphragmatic lobe)

Accessory lobe (intermediate lobe)

Figure 3

Branches of:
Pulmonary vein

Pulmonary artery

Terminal bronchiole

Capillaries in the walls of the alveoli

Alveoli

Urinary System

Kidneys, Ureters, Bladder, and Urethra

PLATE 65

Figure 1. Ventral view of urinary organs and associated organs of the female. For differences in the male cat, see Plate 71.
Figure 2. Frontal section of right kidney.

Color the names and the structures indicated on the plate in the same colors.

Millions of microscopic tubular structures called nephrons are located in the **cortex** and **medulla** of the **kidney**. The urine-producing nephrons are closely associated with the extensive blood supply to the kidney. Collecting ducts extend from nephrons to the **renal crest**, emptying urine into the **pelvis** of the kidney. The pelvis is essentially the beginning of the **ureter**.

Urine is a solution of the products of nitrogen and sulfur metabolism (the processing of substances, mainly nutrients, by the various tissues of the body), Urine also contains inorganic salts, pigments, and the products of toxins inactivated by the liver and excreted by the kidneys. Kidneys regulate the normal levels of substances in the blood such as water, inorganic salts and glucose (blood sugar). In diabetes, the kidneys cannot return excess levels of glucose to the blood, and it spills over into the urine.

Like the nearby **adrenal glands**, kidneys are also endocrine organs. One product regulates blood pressure; another initiates red blood cell production.

Feline urine is watery and yellow. When more water is consumed, urine is diluted and paler. The volume of water excreted varies with water and food consumption, physical activity and environmental temperature. The volume of urine excreted each day is from .03 to 1.6 ounces per pound of body weight.

Urinary calculi (L., pebbles), commonly called kidney and bladder stones or gravel, are abnormal concretions of inorganic salts. They often occur in cats, sometimes occluding the male urethra.

The urinary bladder has two functions:
1. It is a reservoir that expands to contain the urine that is continuously passed to it through the ureters from the kidneys.
2. When a male cat marks his territory, when some cats are frightened, the bladder voids urine. Smooth muscle fibers of the detrusor muscle in the bladder wall contract and the striated muscle in the wall of the urethra relaxes. Neural control of the bladder is complex.

Figure 1

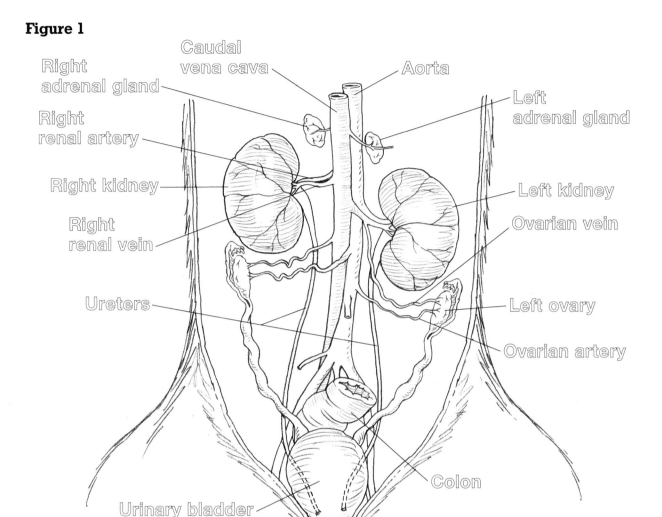

Right adrenal gland
Caudal vena cava
Aorta
Left adrenal gland
Right renal artery
Right kidney
Left kidney
Right renal vein
Ovarian vein
Ureters
Left ovary
Ovarian artery
Colon
Urinary bladder
Urethra

Figure 2

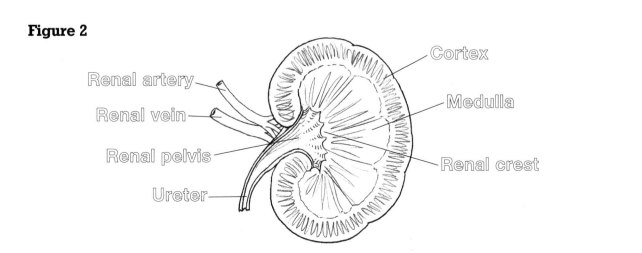

Renal artery
Cortex
Renal vein
Medulla
Renal pelvis
Renal crest
Ureter

Female Reproductive System

Vulva and Vagina

PLATE 66

Figure 1. Caudal view of **perineum** between **anus** and **vulva**. The vulva consists of two **labia** (L., lips) and the **clitoris**. The clitoris is homologous with the penis of the male, and rarely contains a small clitoral bone.

Figure 2. Dorsal view of opened vulva and **vagina** (L., sheath). The **external uterine ostium** of the **cervix** can not be seen, since it faces ventrad. The **bladder** is displaced to one side.

Figure 3. Lateral view of vagina, vulva and related organs. Notice the following:
  • Ventral projection of the cervix into the **fornix** of the vagina.
  • Ventral slope of the caudal vagina and the **vaginal vestibule**.

Using different colors, color the names and the structures indicated.

When a queen is in <u>heat</u> (proestrus and estrus), her labia are swollen and male cats are attracted. The odor of a queen in heat is sensed from quite a distance by the male cat's vomeronasal organs (See Plate 42). During estrus (latter part of heat), when oocytes are discharged from the ovary, the queen will accept mating.

The queen is an <u>induced ovulator</u> (ovulates only if mated). She first enters an estrous cycle around five to seven months of age, and she is a long-day breeder, coming into estrus two to four times a year during the late spring and summer months. The length of each estrous cycle is from 14 to 21 days. The duration of proestrus is from five to seven days; the duration of estrus, from 4 to 13 days. Thus a queen can be in heat for several days. The duration of pregnancy is from 63 to 65 days.

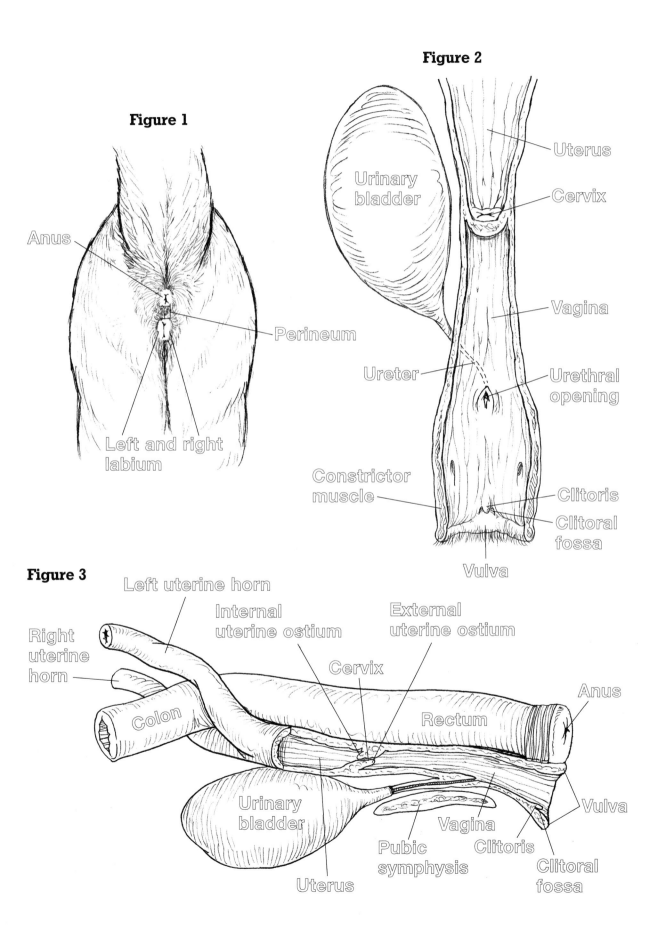

Figure 1

Anus

Perineum

Left and right labium

Figure 2

Urinary bladder

Uterus

Cervix

Vagina

Ureter

Urethral opening

Constrictor muscle

Clitoris

Clitoral fossa

Vulva

Figure 3

Left uterine horn

Internal uterine ostium

External uterine ostium

Cervix

Right uterine horn

Anus

Colon

Rectum

Urinary bladder

Vulva

Uterus

Pubic symphysis

Vagina

Clitoris

Clitoral fossa

Uterus, Uterine Tubes, and Ovaries

PLATE 67

Figure 1. Ventral view of uterus, uterine tubes, ovarian bursae (containing ovaries) and related organs.

The uterus consists of right and left **horns** (L., cornua uteri), **body** (L., corpus uteri) and **neck** (L., cervix uteri). Notice the following: The **left ovarian vein** joins the left renal vein, while the right ovarian vein joins the **caudal caval vein**; the ovarian and uterine vessels anastomose (join together).

Figure 2. The ovarian bursa is part of the mesosalpynx (the peritoneal fold that suspends the uterine tube). It partly encloses the ovary in the queen.

Color the names and the structures indicated in the figures, using different colors.

When a queen is spayed (ovariohysterectomized), an incision is made through the ventral abdominal wall. The **suspensory ligaments of the ovaries** are cut, and the **ovarian arteries** and **veins** are ligated (tied off). The **broad ligament** (mostly mesometrium) is incised longitudinally. **Uterine arteries** and **veins** are ligated along with the body of the uterus which is then crushed and cut cranial to the cervix. The ovaries, uterine tubes and uterus are removed, and the body wall is sutured (sewn) closed.

In Figure 2, notice how close the **ovary** is to the **opening of the uterine tube**. During estrus (in the latter part of heat), oocytes (egg cells) produced by rupture of ovarian follicles are moved into the uterine tube by **fimbriae**, enclosing folds lined with ciliated cells. If spermatozoa (or sperm cells) from the male have made their way to the beginning part of the uterine tube, fertilization (a sperm cell uniting with an oocyte) occurs. A resultant embryo is a ball of dividing cells, a morula. It takes about a week for morulae to pass through the uterine tubes to the cavities of uterine horns.

Figure 1

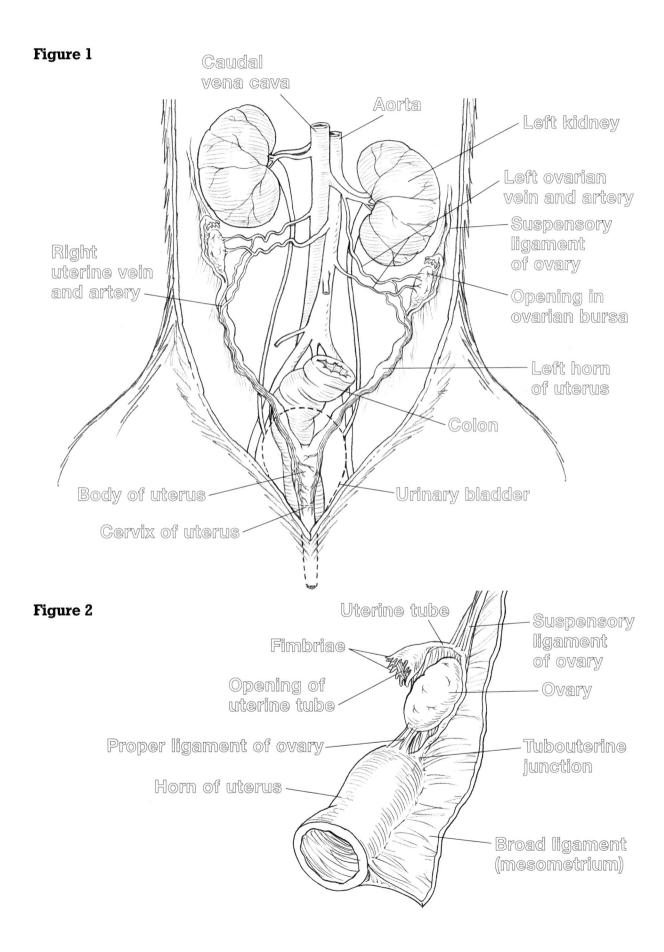

Caudal vena cava

Aorta

Left kidney

Left ovarian vein and artery

Suspensory ligament of ovary

Opening in ovarian bursa

Right uterine vein and artery

Left horn of uterus

Colon

Body of uterus

Urinary bladder

Cervix of uterus

Figure 2

Uterine tube

Fimbriae

Suspensory ligament of ovary

Opening of uterine tube

Ovary

Proper ligament of ovary

Tubouterine junction

Horn of uterus

Broad ligament (mesometrium)

Fetal Membranes and The Placenta

PLATE 68

Figure 1. Sectioned blastula (blastocyst).

Upon arriving in the uterus, each morula develops into a blastula that continues to develop as it floats free in the uterus for another week. The embryos become distributed evenly between the two uterine horns.

In the blastula stage, The **inner cell mass of stem cells** is the early embryo. Cells of the **trophoblast** will form the chorionic epithelium of the chorioallantois. The **zona pellucida**, which surrounded the oocyte, soon disintegrates.

Color names and structures indicated here and in the following figures.

Figure 2. Lateral view of a later embryo and developing extraembryonic membranes. At first and continuing on, the embryo is nourished by blood vessels of the **yolk sac**, the first membrane to grow out from the primitive gut. A remnant of the yolk sac persists until birth. **Chorioamniotic folds** meet and break through, forming the **chorion** and the **amnion** that encloses the amniotic cavity around the **embryo**. The **allantois** grows out (arrows) from the primitive gut and joins the **chorion**, forming the **chorioallantois**. Fluid accumulates in the cavities.

Figure 3. Extraembryonic membranes, zonary placenta and fetus. The process of implantation starts at the end of the free period and lasts a few days. Part of the choroallantois adheres to the endometrium (uterine lining) in a zonary fashion. Chorionic epithelial cells (trophoblast cells) destroy endometrial tissues to come in contact with maternal capillaries. Fetal blood is in the allantoic capillaries of the chorioallantois. This region is the intricate **membranous labyrinth**.

Marginal hematomas along each side are masses of maternal blood. A placenta consists of two parts: fetal and maternal. Transfer of nutrients and oxygen from the mother's blood passes from maternal capillaries and trophoblast cells to fetal capillaries; waste materials and carbon dioxide pass in the opposite direction. Normally, fetal blood and maternal blood never mix.

Figure 4. Feline zonary placenta at term obtained by surgical delivery (Cesarian section). Marginal hematomas now appear reddish brown because of the decomposition of hemglobin. Color names and the structures indicated, using red-brown for the **marginal hematomas** and red for the **membranous labyrinth**. Decomposed hemoglobin is often seen on the fur around the vulva following delivery of kittens.

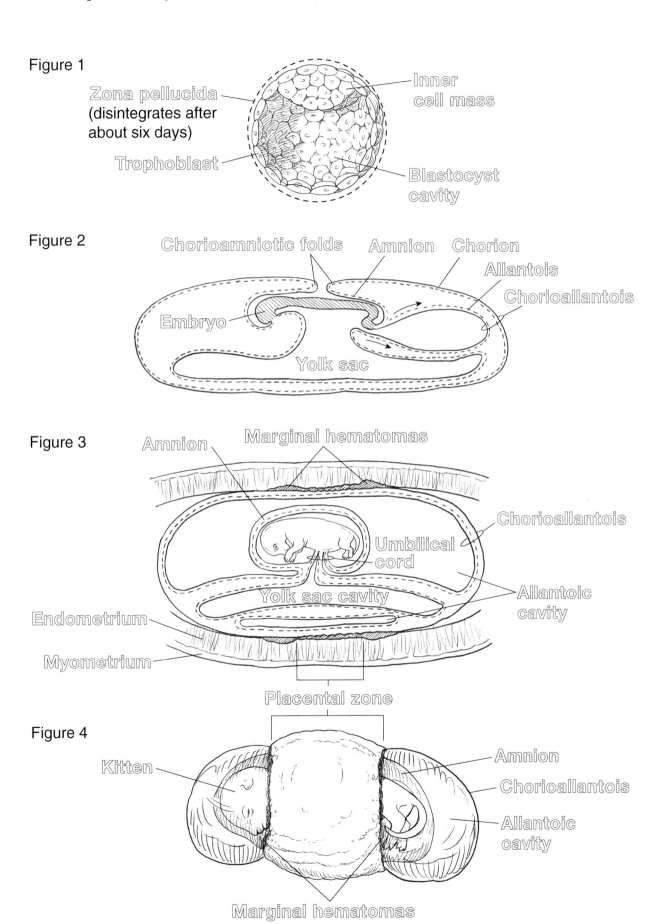

Figure 1

Zona pellucida (disintegrates after about six days)

Inner cell mass

Trophoblast

Blastocyst cavity

Figure 2

Chorioamniotic folds   Amnion   Chorion

Allantois

Chorioallantois

Embryo

Yolk sac

Figure 3

Amnion   Marginal hematomas

Chorioallantois

Umbilical cord

Allantoic cavity

Endometrium

Yolk sac cavity

Myometrium

Placental zone

Figure 4

Kitten

Amnion

Chorioallantois

Allantoic cavity

Marginal hematomas

Parturition

PLATE 69

Figure 1. Cranial presentation of a kitten at delivery. Notice the protrusion of the chorioallantoic sac through the vulva. It is filled with allantoic fluid.

Figure 2. Caudal presentation of a kitten at delivery.

Using different colors, color the names and the structures indicated.

The average length of the <u>gestation period</u> (duration of pregnancy) in the queen is 63 days. Extremes range from 59 to 70 days.

Some signs of impending <u>parturition</u> (the process of giving birth):
- Enlarged abdomen. Usually, but not always, an enlarged, relaxed vulva
- Periodic discharge of clear mucus. Sometimes dried blood left over from the last heat.
- Increased size of mammary glands. Milk may be squeezed from the teats during during the last week of pregnancy.
- Body temperature drops one degree below a physiologic subnormal temperature about 24 hours prior to parturition. Temperature should be taken every 12 hours.

Stage 1 of labor.
 Cervix dilates until it fills the caudal end of the vagina.
 Seclusion and nest building. Poor appetite.
 Increasing discomfort caused by uterine contractions. Rest, change position, walk, etc

Stage 2 of labor - <u>delivery</u> of kittens
 Labor contractions by ventral abdominal muscles create an abdominal press.
 will urinate, have a bowel movement, and possibly vomit.
 Kittens and fetal membranes are moved through the uterus, over the pubic brim and through the birth canal (cervix, vagina and vulva). **Cranial presentation** occurs more commonly than **caudal presentation**.

The **chorioallantoic sac** (long dashes) filled with allantoic fluid emerges through the vulva or it may rupture first. The **amnionic sac** (short dashes) around the kitten will also rupture. These fluids provide lubrication for the passage of the kitten through the vagina. The kitten usually does not require assistance in delivery. With continuous licking, the queen will rupture any intact fetal membranes and remove them from the kitten.

Expulsion of the placenta.
 The queen pulls on the membranes and umbilical cord, pulling the placenta out. There is some bleeding. The feline placenta is <u>deciduate</u>, that is, there is some loss of maternal tissue (mostly blood) at birth. The queen eats the fetal membranes and placenta.

<u>Cesarian section</u> (C-section), surgical delivery, is indicated when kittens are too large to pass through the pelvic opening or when they are in a position that prevents their passage from the uterus and through the birth canal.

Figure 1

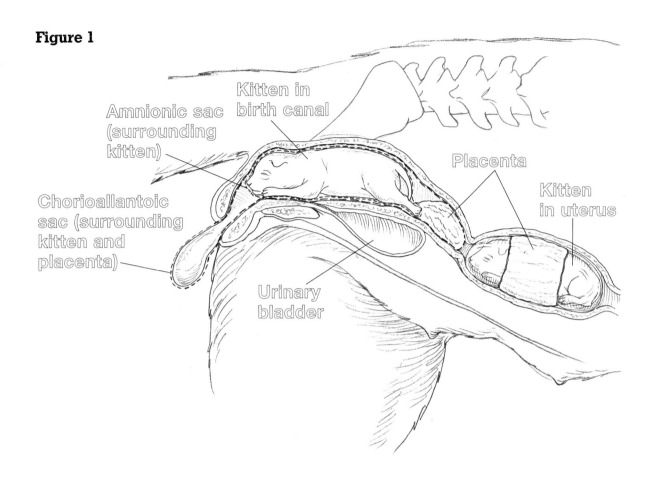

Amnionic sac (surrounding kitten)

Kitten in birth canal

Placenta

Kitten in uterus

Chorioallantoic sac (surrounding kitten and placenta)

Urinary bladder

Figure 2

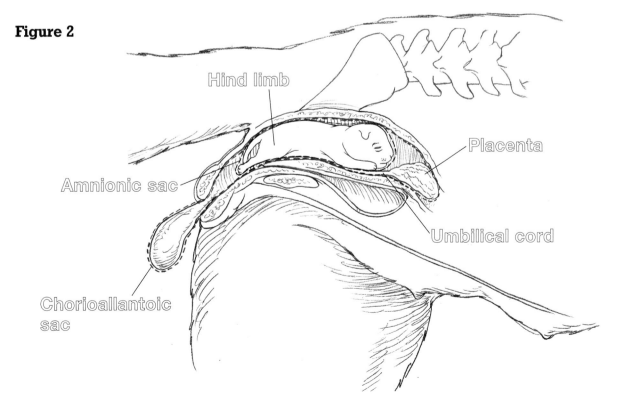

Hind limb

Placenta

Amnionic sac

Umbilical cord

Chorioallantoic sac

Feline Mammary Glands

PLATE 70

Figure 1. Ventral view of feline mammary glands
Figure 2. Diagrammatic drawing of a feline mammary gland.

Using different colors, color the names and the structures indicated.

There may be four (usually) to six pairs of mammary glands, but glands may be missing on either side. Frequently, opposite glands may be slightly staggered. This is a beneficial arrangement, since it provides better access for nursing kittens.

Mammary glands are modified sweat glands that develop to produce milk (lactate). **Secretory cells** lining **tubuloalveoli** produce milk. Star-shaped **contractile cells** (myoepithelial cells) surround each tubuloalveolus, **Lactiferous ducts** carry milk to **lactiferous sinuses**. Several **papillary ducts** (teat canals) open on the end of the teat.

The skin of the teat is covered with fine hairs.

Late in pregnancy, mammary glands become larger as the secretory cells produce more and more milk. In the final week or ten days, milk can be squeezed from the teats. The enlarged glands droop down, and opposite glands may touch one another.

All of the mammary glands lactate. When kittens begin to suckle (nurse), the mammary glands adjust to accommodate the number of kittens in the litter. Unneeded glands become swollen and firm, but the swelling soon decreases. Normally lactating glands become swollen and then decrease in size as they are suckled.

Suckling starts the "let-down reflex". Nervous stimulation by suckling causes secretion of a hormone (oxytocin from the pituitary gland). Oxytocin stimulates contractile cells around the tubuloalveoli to squeeze milk out into the lactiferous ducts.

The first milk produced, colostrum, has a laxative effect on the kittens. Colostrum also contains important antibodies that are ingested by the newborn kitten during the first day of its life. These antibodies provide protection against diseases for several weeks.

A firm, swollen, warm, possibly red mammary gland indicates mastitis, inflammation of a mammary gland caused by bacterial infection. Milk squeezed from the gland may have the thick appearance of pus, or it may be blood-streaked. A veterinarian should be consulted.

Mammary gland tumors, many cancerous, can occur in cats. Lymph drainage from the cranial three glands on each side goes to the axillary lymph node; lymph drainage from the caudal two glands goes to the superficial inguinal lymph node.

Figure 1

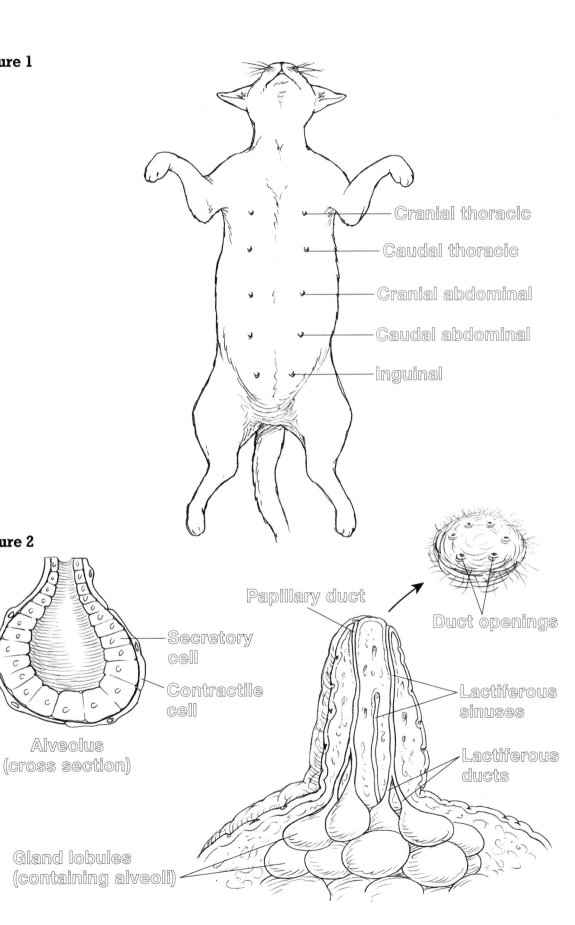

Cranial thoracic

Caudal thoracic

Cranial abdominal

Caudal abdominal

Inguinal

Figure 2

Papillary duct

Duct openings

Secretory cell

Contractile cell

Lactiferous sinuses

Lactiferous ducts

Alveolus (cross section)

Gland lobules (containing alveoli)

Male Reproductive System

Male Genital Organs

PLATE 71

Figure 1. Diagrammatic drawing of the male genital organs. Left lateral view.
Color the **boldfaced names** below and color the structures indicated on the plate.

1. **Deferent duct**
2. **Ureter**
3. **Bladder**
4. **Testicular vessels**
5. **Spermatic cord** (within inguinal canal)
6. **Prepuce**
7. **Body of the penis**
8. **Glans penis**
9. **Scrotum**
10. **Testis**

11. **Vaginal tunic**
12. **Rectum**
13. **Pubic bone**
14. **Ventral abdominal wall**
15. **Left gracilis m.**
16. **Bulbospongious m.**
17. **Penile retractor muscle**
18. **Bulbourethral gland**
19. **Urethra**
20. **Prostate**

Figure 2. Section of right testis and epididymis. Color the names and the structures indicated in different colors.

Each **testis** (Latin), (English, testicle; Greek, orchis) is suspended by a fold of peritoneum, the mesorchium, and enclosed by its continuaton, the **vaginal tunic**. Deep to the visceral part of the vaginal tunic, the dense fibrous connnective tissue **tunica albuginea** and its internally projecting septula support the testis. The **scrotum** is a pouch of skin, smooth muscle, fascia and parietal vaginal tunic. The space between the visceral and parietal parts of the vaginal tunic is actually peritoneal cavity. Muscle in the scrotum and the cremaster muscles in the spermatic cord assist in regulating the temperature of the testicles by raising and lowering them from the body wall.

Spermatozoa (sperm cells) develop in **seminiferous tubules**. They pass through **straight tubules, testicular rete** (L., network) and **efferent ductules** into the **epididymal duct** in the **head of the epididymis**. As spermatozoa pass through the epididymal duct, they mature under the influence of secretions from the cells lining the duct. The terminal part of the epididymal duct in the **tail of the epididymis** and the first part of the **deferent duct** contain mature, moderately motile spermatozoa with whip-like tails. The very muscular (smooth muscle) deferent duct continues up in the **spermatic cord** through the inguinal canal and terminates by opening into the prostatic part of the pelvic **urethra**. During ejaculation, each deferent duct propels spermatozoa and epididymal fluid to the urethra.

Figure 1

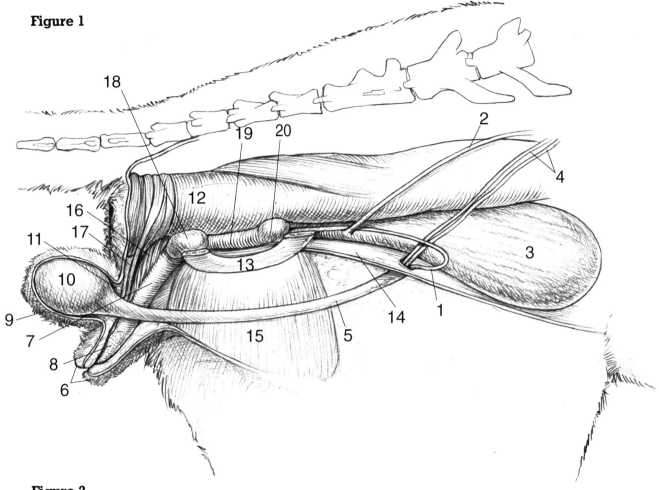

Figure 2

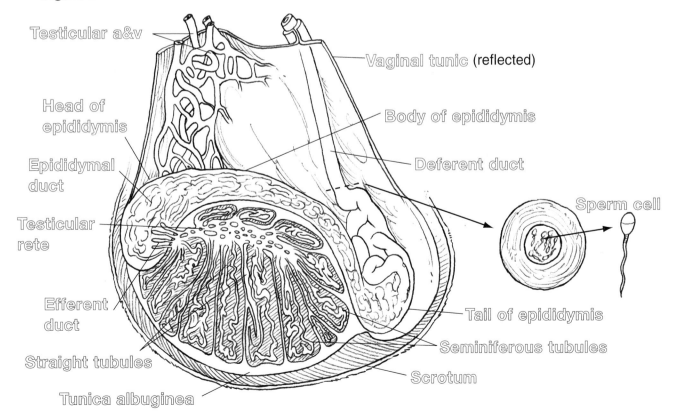

Testicular a&v

Vaginal tunic (reflected)

Head of
epididymis

Body of epididymis

Epididymal
duct

Deferent duct

Testicular
rete

Sperm cell

Efferent
duct

Tail of epididymis

Straight tubules

Seminiferous tubules

Scrotum

Tunica albuginea

Prostate, Bulbourethral Gland, Penis

PLATE 72

Figure 1. Prostate. A. Dorsal view. B. Ventral view with urethra opened.
Figure 2. Relations of the erectile tissue bodies of the feline penis: roots of the penis, cavernous bodies, bulb of the penis, spongy body of the urethra, spongy body of the penile glans (L., glans penis)
Figure 3. A. Isolated penile bone (L., os penis. also termed <u>baculum</u>).
       B. Cross section of bulb of glans penis

Color the names and structures indicated on the drawings.

The **prostate** and the **bulbourethral gland** are the accessory sex glands in the cat. Right and left lobes of the prostate gland partially enclose the prostatic part of the **urethra**. Numerous ducts from secretory glandular units enter the urethra as it passes through the gland.

At the time of ejaculation, a mass of sperm cells and epididymal fluid is moved by muscular contractions of the **deferent ducts** and **ischiocavernous muscles** to the slit-like openings of the deferent ducts on each side of the **seminal hillock** in the dorsal wall of the prostatic urethra. This mass is moved toward the external urethral opening by contractions of the **urethral** and **bulbospongious muscles**. Then the prostate secretes, and the prostatic fluid and fluid from urethral glands is moved out, completing the formation of <u>semen</u>.

The two **roots** (or crura, L., legs) **of the penis** originate on the ischiatic tubers covered by the **ischiocavernous muscles**. They continue into the two **cavernous bodies** in the body of the penis. The **bulb of the penis** is situated between the two roots. It continues into the **spongy body of the urethra**. This expands into the **spongy body of the glans**. Arteries and veins of the penis are terminal branches of the internal pudendal vessels.

Erection of the penis is brought about by the complete filling of the erectile tissue bodies with blood. The male bites the back of the queen's neck, mounts and thrusts. A complex sequence of arterial relaxation and interference with venous drainage caused by contractions of the muscles around the penis and the muscle of the vagina, these thrusts, direct the urethral opening of the penis up toward the external opening of the cervix.

At the end of intercourse, arterial flow returns to normal and muscles relax, permitting veins to open fully. The two **penile retractor muscles** contract, assisting the return of the penile glans into the **prepuce**.

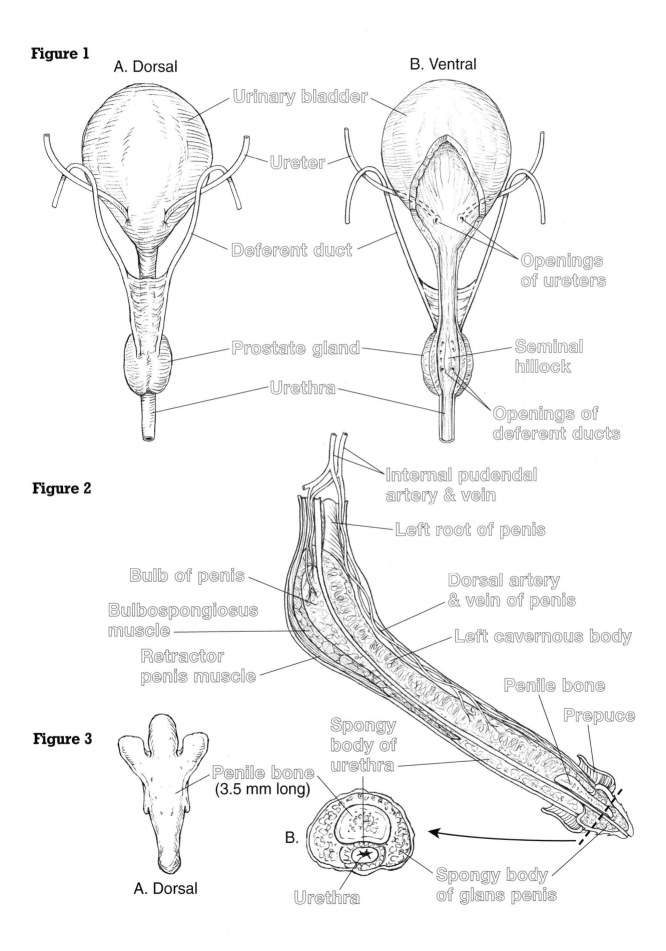

Figure 1

A. Dorsal

B. Ventral

Urinary bladder

Ureter

Deferent duct

Openings
of ureters

Seminal
hillock

Prostate gland

Openings of
deferent ducts

Urethra

Figure 2

Internal pudendal
artery & vein

Left root of penis

Bulb of penis

Dorsal artery
& vein of penis

Bulbospongiosus
muscle

Left cavernous body

Retractor
penis muscle

Penile bone

Prepuce

Figure 3

Penile bone
(3.5 mm long)

Spongy
body of
urethra

B.

Spongy body
of glans penis

A. Dorsal

Urethra

Descent of the Testes

PLATE 73

Diagrammatic drawings:
Figure 1. Testis and epididymis prior to entering inguinal canal. Extra-abdominal part of the gubernaculum increases in volume to enlarge the inguinal canal and scrotum.
Figure 2. Loop formed by the epididymis and deferent duct enters expanded inguinal canal first.
Figure 3. Testis and epididymis within the scrotum. Remnant of the gubernaculum persists as the ligament of the tail of the epididymis and proper ligament of the testis (not seen here). The parietal vaginal tunic (from the vaginal process) lines the scrotum; the visceral vaginal tunic covers the testis and epididymis.

Using different colors, color the names and structures indicated.

Each **testis** (plural = testes) begins as a swelling under a temporary middle kidney. As the developing testis begins to descend, the middle kidney regresses, but its duct becomes the **duct of the epididymis** and the **deferent duct**.

The **inguinal canal** is a potential space between the internal abdominal oblique muscle and the fibrous aponeurosis of the external abdominal oblique muscle. A slit in the aponeurosis is the superficial inguinal ring. The **gubernaculum** (L., helm) of jelly-like embryonic tissue (mesenchyme) grows and swells, expanding the **vaginal ring**, the inguinal canal and finally the **scrotum**. The descent of the testes is passive, forced by pressure from the growing organs around them. The gubernaculum is only a guide and does not contract even as it regresses. As the testis and epididymis descend into the **vaginal process**, they are covered with the inner **visceral vaginal tunic** that becomes continuous with the mesorchium (peritoneum suspending the testis). As each testis enters its compartment of the scrotum, the soft, regressing gubernaculum changes to the short, fibrous proper ligament of the testis between the testis and the epididymis and **ligament of tail of epididymis** that connects with the connective tissue of the scrotum.

The descent of the testes occurs in the last part of pregnancy and first several days after birth. The stimulus for descent of the testes is the hormone, testosterone, produced by cells within the testes. The testes are normally at the vaginal ring or into the inguinal canal at the time of birth. They should be completely descended into the scrotum by two weeks after birth. Due to the small size of the immature testes, they usually cannot be felt from the exterior until around six weeks after birth.

Retained testicle or cryptorchidism (Gr., kryptos, hidden, orchis, testis) can occur in cats. The cryptorchid testis may be under the skin of the flank between the superficial inguinal ring and the scrotum. Two other locations are the inguinal canal or the abdominal cavity. Because of higher temperature, a retained testicle cannot produce spermatozoa, although it can still produce the hormone, testosterone. A monorchid (only one descended testicle) cat should not be used for breeding, since the abnormality is considered heritable.

Figure 1

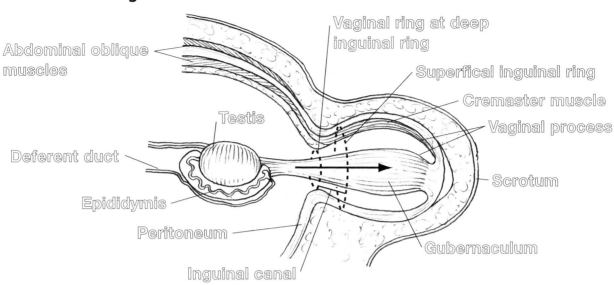

Abdominal oblique muscles

Deferent duct

Testis

Epididymis

Peritoneum

Inguinal canal

Vaginal ring at deep inguinal ring

Superfical inguinal ring

Cremaster muscle

Vaginal process

Scrotum

Gubernaculum

Figure 2

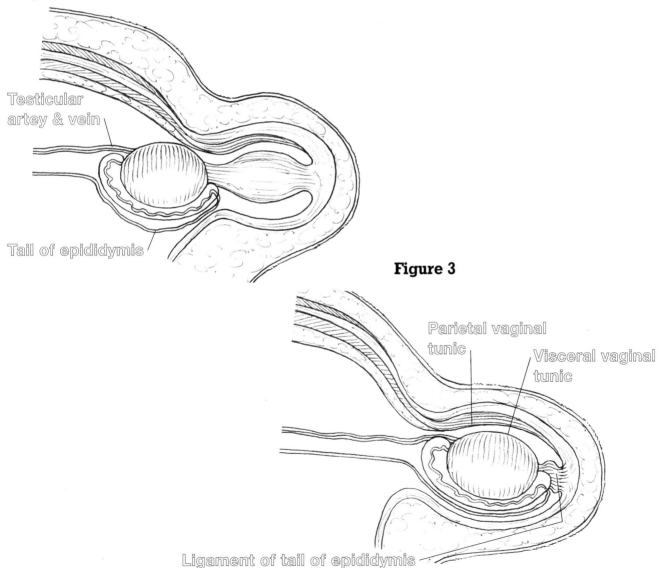

Testicular artey & vein

Tail of epididymis

Figure 3

Parietal vaginal tunic

Visceral vaginal tunic

Ligament of tail of epididymis

Nervous System

The Brain

PLATE 74

Figure 1. Dorsal view of brain.
Figure 2. Median section of brain.

Using different colors, underline the **boldfaced names** below and color structures indicated on the plate.

1. **Longitudinal fissure**
2. **Right cerebral hemisphere**
3. **Sulci** (grooves)
4. **Gyri** (convolutions)
5. **Cerebellum**
6. **Corpus callosum** (connects cerebral hemispheres)
7. **Septum pellucidum**
8. **Pineal gland**
9. **Medulla oblongata**
10. **Pons**
11. **Thalamus**
12. **Hypothalamus**
13. **Hypophysis cerebri** (pituitary gland)
14. **Optic chiasm**
15. **Olfactory bulb**

The hypothalamus, hypophysis cerebri and pineal gland are parts of the endocrine system.

The three large parts of the brain are the cerebrum (with its two hemispheres), brain stem and cerebellum. The brain stem consists of the pons, medulla oblongata, midbrain (mesencephalon) and diencephalon. The brain stem connects the cerebral hemispheres with the cerebellum and the spinal cord.

Figure 1

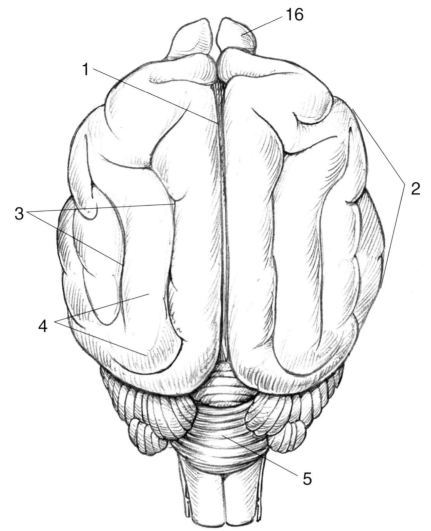

Figure 2

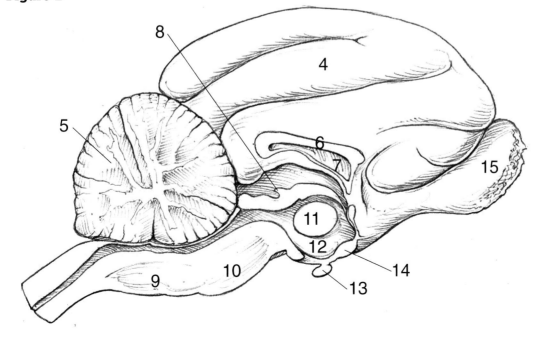

Cranial Nerves

PLATE 75

Ventral view of brain and cranial nerve roots.

In different colors, color the Roman numerals and the cranial nerves indicated on the plate.

CRANIAL NERVES   FUNCTIONS

I. Olfactory nerve - Sense of smell. Many small nerve fibers come from the mucous membrane of the two nasal fossae. They pass through openings in the cribriform plate of the ethmoid bone to the **olfactory bulbs**.

II. Optic nerve - Vision. Some nerve fibers coming from the retina of one eye cross over at the **optic chiasm** and continue into the optic tract of the opposite side.

III. Oculomotor nerve - Motor to several skeletal muscles around the eye. Parasympathetic fibers motor to smooth muscles within the eye.

IV. Trochlear nerve - Motor to dorsal oblique muscle around the eye.

V. Trigeminal nerve - Sensory to face. Motor to muscles of mastication (chewing) and deep muscles of the head. Sensory to lower teeth. Lingual branch sensory for touch to the tongue.

VI. Abducent nerve - Motor to two skeletal muscles around the eye.

VII. Facial nerve - Motor to facial, eyelid and ear muscles. Its chorda tympani branch joins the lingual nerve and senses taste from the rostral 2/3 of the tongue. Parasympathetic fibers are motor to lacrimal and salivary glands.

VIII. Vestibulocochlear nerve - Sensory for hearing and for motion and balance.

IX. Glossopharyngeal nerve - Motor to skeletal muscles of palate and pharynx. Senses taste from the caudal 1/3 of tongue. Sensory to mucous membrane of palate and pharynx. Pararsympathetic fibers to salivary glands.

X. Vagus nerve - Parasympathetic nerves to smooth muscle and glands of cervical, thoracic and abdominal viscera. Sensory to external ear. Sensory to laryngeal mucous membrane and motor to laryngeal muscles via cranial and caudal laryngeal nerves.

XI. Accessory nerve - Motor to four shoulder muscles. Notice the main part of the nerve coming from the cervical spinal cord.

XII. Hypoglossal nerve - Motor to muscles of the tongue.

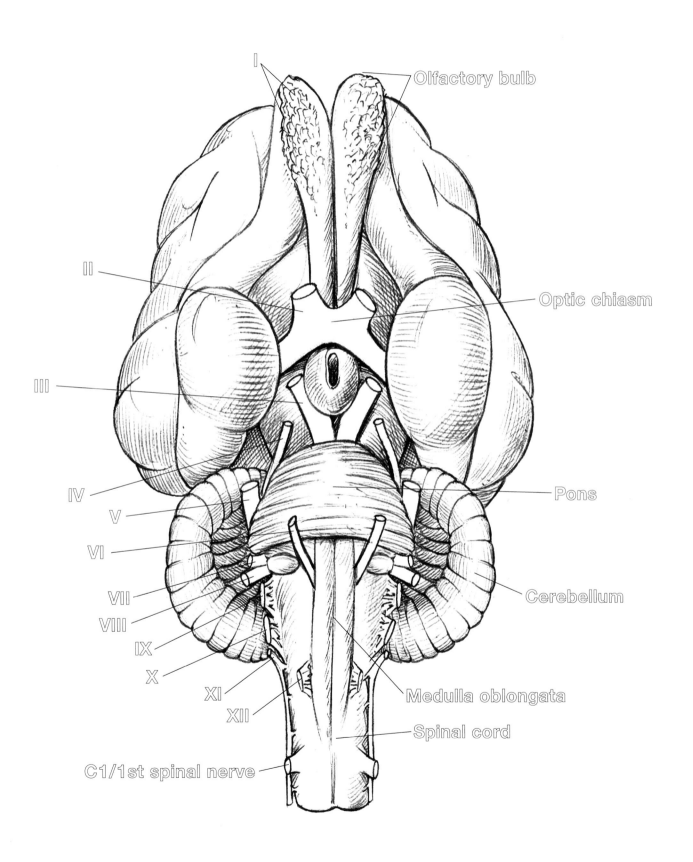

I
Olfactory bulb

II
Optic chiasm

III

IV

V

VI

VII

VIII

IX

X

XI

XII

Pons

Cerebellum

Medulla oblongata

Spinal cord

C1/1st spinal nerve

Spinal Cord and Spinal Nerves

PLATE 76

Figure 1. Diagrammatic dorsal view of spinal cord and spinal nerve roots.
Using different colors, color the names and the regions of the spinal cord.
Figure 2. Cross section of thoracic region of spinal cord and its relations to the vertebral canal and spinal nerve parts.

Underline **boldfaced names** below in different colors and color indicated structures on the drawing the same colors.

1. **Epidural space** (of vertebral canal)
2. **Dura mater**
3. **Spinal cord**
4. **Dorsal root of spinal nerve** (to and from sympathetic trunk)
5. **Spinal (dorsal root) ganglion**

6. **Ventral root of spinal nerve**
7. **Thoracic spinal nerve**
8. **Communicating branches**
9. **Sympathetic trunk** (Nerve cell bodies and processes)

The spinal cord continues from the medulla oblongata at the <u>foramen magnum</u> of the occipital bone, extending caudad to around the level of the intervertebral disc between L6 and L7. Differential development accounts for the presence of an eighth cervical spinal cord segment and variable relations of spinal cord segments to vertebrae. Caudal lumbar, sacral and caudal segments of the cord lie more and more cranial to vertebrae of the same number.

The **cauda equina** (L., horse's tail) is the collection of spinal nerve roots that extend caudad from the end of the spinal cord within the vertebral canal.

The diameter of the spinal cord is greatest at the **cervical** and **lumbar enlargements** where the nerve roots for the plexuses supplying the nerves of the limbs originate.

A <u>sensory</u> **dorsal root** (with its **spinal ganglion**) and a <u>motor</u> **ventral root** join to form a **spinal nerve**. The spinal nerve then divides into major <u>dorsal and ventral branches</u>. In the **thoracic** and **lumbar regions, communicating branches** connect with the **sympathetic trunk**.The latter is formed by a series of <u>ganglia connected by nerves</u>. lying along the inner surface of the thoracic wall.

The <u>dura mater,</u> outermost meninx covering the spinal cord, is separated from the wall of the vertebral canal by an <u>epidural space</u>. This space contains some fatty tissue and a venous plexus. Spinal nerves pass through the meninges.

Figure 1

Figure 2

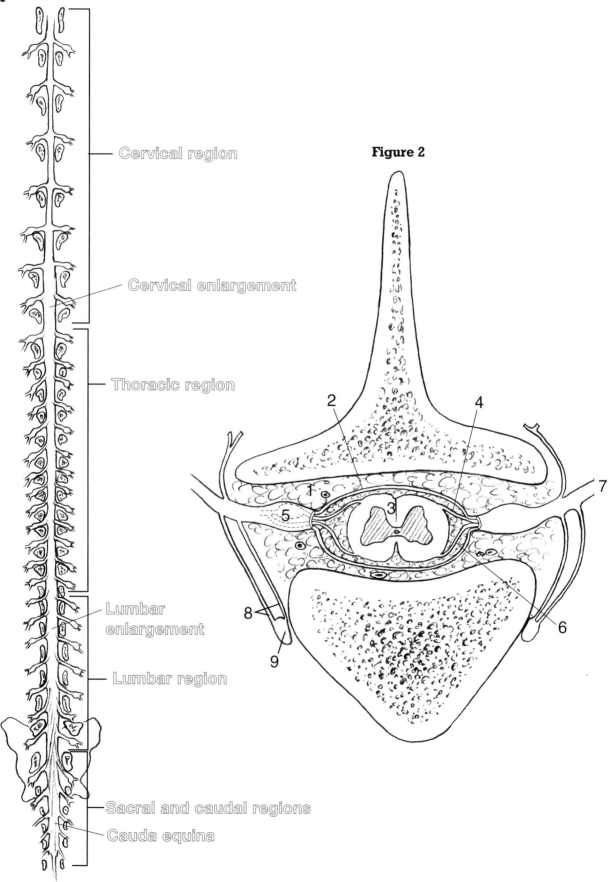

Cervical region

Cervical enlargement

Thoracic region

Lumbar enlargement

Lumbar region

Sacral and caudal regions

Cauda equina

2

4

1

3

5

7

6

8

9

Autonomic Nervous System

PLATE 77

Color the parts of the SYMPATHETIC DIVISION of the ANS red.
1. Thoracolumbar region of the the spinal cord ("thoracolumbar outflow")
2. Paravertebral, cervical and prevertebral ganglia
3. Postganglionic and some sensory connecting nerves to cephalic, thoracic, abdominal and pelvic viscera and skin.

Color the parts of the PARASYMPATHETIC DIVISION of the ANS blue.
1. Cranial region (of the "craniosacral outflow") in the medulla oblongata
   Nuclei of cranial nerves III, VII, IX and X (long vagus nerve)
   Ganglia of cranial nerves III, VII, IX and X
   Intramural ganglia of vagus nerve in the myenteric plexus
2. Sacral region of the (of the "craniosacral outflow")
   Pelvic nerve and ganglia

Most common neurotransmitters released by ANS neurons:
1. Preganglionic neurons - acetylcholine. Released in ganglia
2. Postganglionic neurons
   Sympathetic - norepinephrine - effector
   Parasympathetic - acetylcholine - effector

Effectors: smooth muscle, cardiac muscle, glands

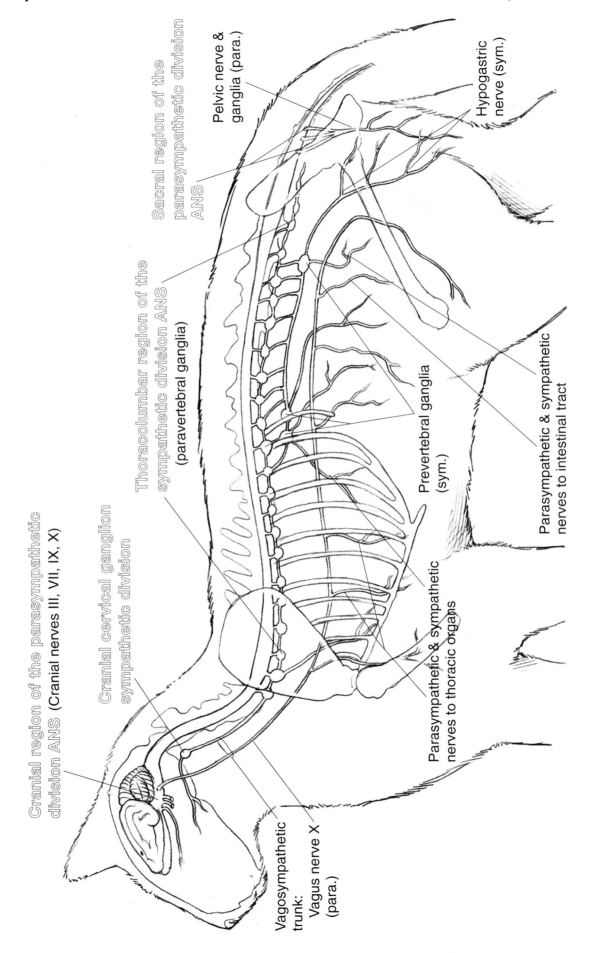

Cranial region of the parasympathetic
division ANS (Cranial nerves III, VII, IX, X)

Cranial cervical ganglion
sympathetic division

Thoracolumbar region of the
sympathetic division ANS
(paravertebral ganglia)

Sacral region of the
parasympathetic division
ANS

Pelvic nerve &
ganglia (para.)

Hypogastric
nerve (sym.)

Prevertebral ganglia
(sym.)

Parasympathetic & sympathetic
nerves to intestinal tract

Parasympathetic & sympathetic
nerves to thoracic organs

Vagosympathetic
trunk:
Vagus nerve X
(para.)

Central and Peripheral Nervous Systems

PLATE 78

The central nervous system consists of the cerebrum, mesencephalon, cerebellum, brainstem, and the spinal cord. The peripheral (somatic) nervous system consists of the 12 cranial nerves, 31 pairs of spinal nerves with dorsal and ventral rami, and the autonomic nervous system (plate 77). The ventral rami form the plexuses; cervical, brachial, lumbar, and sacral, these in turn give off most of the major nerves of the body outside of the 12 cranial nerves. The dorsal rami in general give off individual nerves to the back and trunk.

Central nervous system:
1. Olfactory bulb
2. Cerebrum
3. Cerebellum
4. Spinal cord
5. Brachial plexus

Somatic (peripheral) nervous system:
6. Thoracic spinal nerves
7. Lumbar spinal nerves
8. Lumbosacral plexus
9. Perineal n.
10. Pudendal n.
11. Obturator n.
12. Sciatic n.
13. Caudal cutaneous femoral n.
14. Caudal cutaneous sural n.
15. Tibial n.
16. Lateral cutaneous n.
17. Medial and lateral plantar nn.
18. Deep fibular n.

19. Superficial fibular n.
20. Common fibular n.
21. Femoral n.
22. Medial and lateral palmar nn.
23. Dorsal common digital n.
24. Superficial br. Radial n.
25. Dorsal common digital n.
26. Ulnar n.
27. Median n.
28. Radial n.
29. Axillary n.
30. Musculocutaneous n.
31. Suprascapular n.

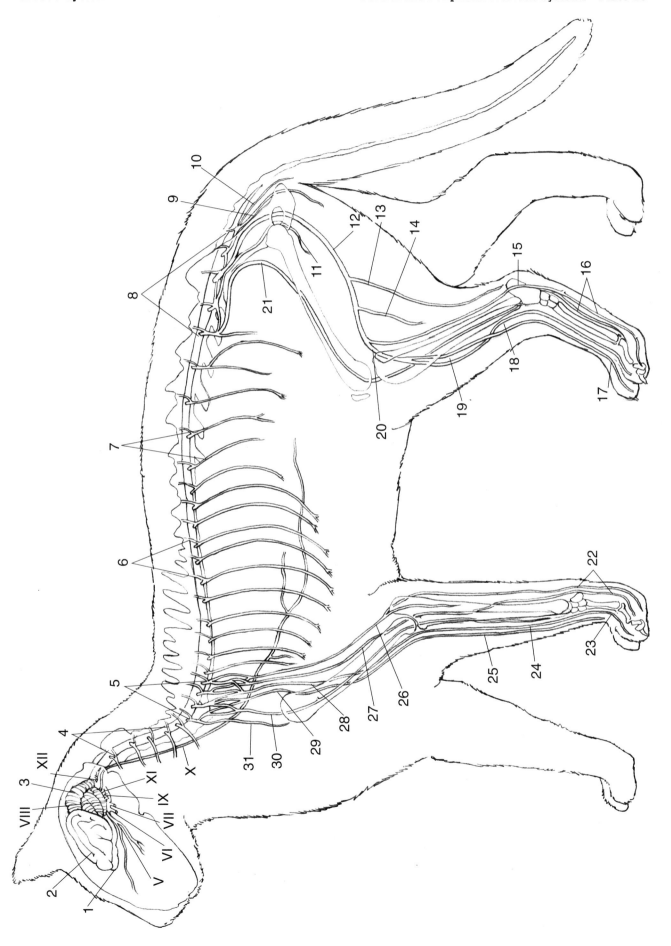

Meninges and Cerebrospinal Fluid System

PLATE 79

Schematic drawing showing:

- Meninges (singular, meninx) - three membranes covering the brain and spinal cord.
- Main sites of production of cerebrospinal fluid (CSF), the **choroid plexuses.**
- CSF is also produced by the lining of the ventricles and brain tissue.
- Circulation of CSF (arrows) through the **ventricles** (communicating chambers of the brain), the central canal of the spinal cord and the **subarachnoid space.**
- Drainage of CSF through projecting **arachnoid granulations** into blood of a **venous sinus** within the **dura mater.**
- End of spinal cord and the **cauda equina** (L., horse's tail) formed by the last few spinal nerves.
- Sites for withdrawal of CSF (A) from the subarachnoid space and for injection of anesthetic into the **epidural space** (B), providing epidural anesthesia.

Underline the **boldfaced terms** in different colors and color the structures indicated by labels

1. **Dura mater of cranial cavity** - blends with periosteum of cranial cavity; no epidural space.
2. **Dura mater of vertebral canal** - dense, fibrous outer meninx.
3. **Epidural space** (only in vertebral canal) - contains adipose tissue, vessels and nerve roots.
4. **Periosteum of vertebral canal**
5. **Arachnoid membrane** - delicate vascular middle meninx.
6. **Subarachnoid space** (greatly enlarged here) - contains CSF. Crossed by spider web-like filaments extending from arachnoid membrane to pia mater.
7. **Pia mater** - vascular inner membrane covering brain and spinal cord; forms terminal filament at end of spinal cord.
8. **Cerebellomedullary cistern** (cisterna magna) - enlarged part of subarachnoid space; site for obtaining a sample of CSF.

9. **Interventricular foramen** (opening) - one each side; connects lateral ventricle in cerebral hemisphere with third ventricle.
10. **Third ventricle** - within midbrain
11. **Choroid plexus of third ventricle** (Choroid plexus of lateral ventricle not seen here.)
12. **Fourth ventricle** - within medulla oblongata
13. **Central canal of spinal cord** - continues caudad from fourth ventricle
14. **Choroid plexus of fourth ventricle**
15. **Lateral aperture of fourth ventricle** - one of three exit foramina for CSF passing into subarachnoid space.
16. **Arachnoid granulations** - through which CSF passes into dorsal sagittal venous sinus.
17. **Dorsal sagittal venous sinus** - within dura mater

CSF functions: 1. Cushions brain and spinal cord. 2. Transports nutrients, waste products and regulatory substances. Hydrocephalus is an expansion of the ventricles filled with an excessive amount of CSF, exerting compression on the brain.

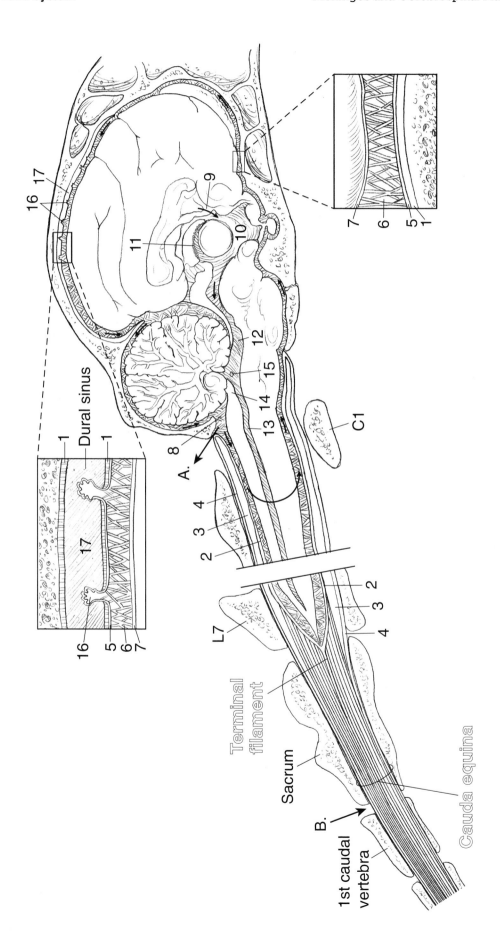

7
6
5
1

16 17

9

11

10

12

13 14 15

C1

8

A.

3 4

2

2
3

4

L7

Terminal filament

Sacrum

B.

1st caudal vertebra

Cauda equina

1
Dural sinus
1

17

16
5
6
7

Endocrine System

Locations of Major Endocrine Organs

PLATE 80

In different colors, underline the **boldfaced names** of the endocrine organs listed and color the organs indicated on the plate.

ENDOCRINE ORGANS	HORMONES PRODUCED	TARGET ORGANS/TISSUES
1. Pineal gland	Melatonin	Sleep centers in brain
2. Hypothalamus	Releasing hormones	Hypophysis cerebri
	Oxytocin	Uterus, mammary glands
	Antidiuretic hormone (ADH)	Kidneys
3. Hypophysis cerebri (pituitary gland)		
Adenohypophysis	Thyrotropin	Thyroid gland
	Gonadotropins	Gonads: ovaries, testes
	Adrenocorticotropin	Adrenal cortices
	Somatotropin	Body's growing tissues
Neurohypophysis	Synthesizes & releases	Oxytocin - mammary gland, uterus
	oxytocin & antediuretic hormone (ADH)	ADH - kidneys
4. Thyroid gland - Two lobes	Tetraiodothyronine & triiodothyronine	All tissues of body
NOT connected by an isthmus in the cat	Calcitonin	Bone
5. Parathyroid glands - two on each side	Parathyroid hormone (PTH)	Bone, intestines, kidneys
6. Thymus	Thymosin	T-lymphocytes
7. Right atrium	Atrial natriuretic peptide (ANP)	Kidney
8. Stomach	Gastrin	Stomach, small intestine
9. Pancreas	Glucagon	All tissues of body
Pancreatic islets	Insulin	All tissues of body
10. Small intestine	Cholecystokinin; secretin	Gall bladder, small intestine
11. Adrenal glands - cortex	Aldosterone, cortisol	All tissues of body, immune organs
- medulla	Epinephrine, norepinephrine	Muscular tissues, glands
12. Ovaries	Estrogens, progesterone	Female reproductive organs
Testes	Testosterone	Male repro. organs, muscle, skin

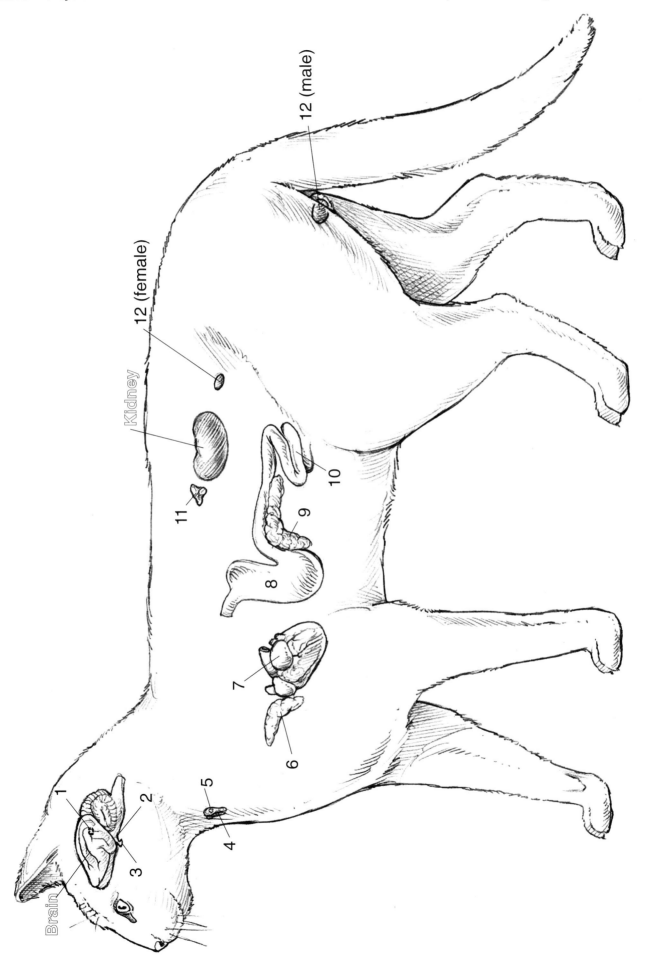

Index

Feline Anatomy - A Coloring Atlas

X

Y

Z